A BODY
MADE
OF GLASS

Also by Caroline Crampton

The Way to the Sea:
The Forgotten Histories of the Thames Estuary

A BODY MADE OF GLASS

A History of Hypochondria

CAROLINE CRAMPTON

GRANTA

Granta Publications, 12 Addison Avenue, London W11 4QR

First published in Great Britain by Granta Books, 2024

Extracts from the following works by Philip Larkin are
reproduced with permission from Faber and Faber Ltd:
'Dockery and Son' and 'Ambulances' in *The Whitsun Weddings;
Letters to Monica*, edited by Anthony Thwaite.

Lines by Philip Larkin and Andrew Motion from *Philip
Larkin: A Writer's Life* by Andrew Motion are reproduced
with permission from Faber and Faber Ltd.

A CIP catalogue record for this book
is available from the British Library.

3 5 7 9 10 8 6 4 2

ISBN 978 1 78378 905 4 (hardback)
ISBN 978 1 78378 507 8 (ebook)

Typeset in Caslon by M Rules

Printed and bound by CPI Group (UK) Ltd, Croydon, CR0 4YY

www.granta.com

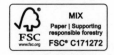

For Guy, the cure to my ailments.

Contents

The rhythms of this ritual are deeply ingrained. Lean forward, closer to the mirror, bracing hips against the sink. Old bruises accepting the hard angles. One hand to pull my shirt away from my left collarbone. The other to poke and prod the shadow I saw there.

It's very bright in the deserted bathroom at work. The overhead strip lighting bounces off the walls, the tiled floor, the gleaming white of the sink and toilet. In the mirror, the room behind me is blanched out of sight. All that is in focus is my own pale face and pinpricked pupils. Blotchy redness is rising out of my collar and climbing up my throat. Turning my head slightly, I avoid catching my own eye in the reflection.

My gaze drops to the two square inches of skin on my neck to the left of my Adam's apple. This is the part of my body that most often flares into quivering sensation, and thus the part I know best. I could reconstruct it perfectly through touch alone, my fingertips following the baseline of the long-healed scar that snakes along parallel with my collarbone and the squashy dips between the tendons running down my neck. But now, I want to see it, to scrutinise it as if through a microscope.

I know the pattern. On bad days, when I'm tired and slow and the quick-fire cross talk of my colleagues washes against my ears like jagged waves of sound, I will turn my head to avoid someone's gaze and feel it. The sensation of something soft and yet hard at the same time catching on the usually smooth mechanism of my pivoting neck. A feeling at once horribly familiar and completely alien. It's like going downstairs in the dark and miscounting so that your foot connects suddenly with the floor when it was expecting to keep on passing downwards through the clear air to another step. A sudden jolt and an electric pulse ripping through the stomach. An intruder is detected.

I know the pattern but can still be stuck in it. I'm pretending to sit at my desk and type normally, but I'm actually listening to the roar of panic in my ears while conducting a fierce argument with myself. It keeps revolving, a sing-song, meaningless wrangle. *You know it's not real | but this time it might be real.* The outcome is always the same. I always end up here, in front of this mirror, staring at this glassy, reflected version of me, quietly weeping and poking myself in the neck hard enough to leave marks.

What my questing fingers are looking for is evidence of a lump, a bulge of flesh that shouldn't be pushing its way out of my neck and yet, somehow, is. Except I can't put it that clearly in my own mind; all there is inside my head as I search is blistering static and a dogged whisper of *it can't be it can't be.* Tumours have a certain texture, I've learned: a hard kernel moored deep inside with a slippery casing that can move over muscle and under skin. When I found one in this part of my neck before, nearly a decade ago, I could roll it between my fingers. It danced across the sinews as I moved my head. It made a clicking sound I could hear with my tongue.

While I'm still poking and staring, my brain wakes up and thoughts start to accelerate away from me. If there really is something growing in my neck – all the images in my mind are fairy-tale malevolence, poisonous yet invisible roses creeping through my flesh to bind my life with their thorny tangles – my existence will be forever changed by it. I will have to deliver the bad news to my husband, my parents, my sister, my friends; navigate the peculiarly modern dilemma of deciding how much of a highly personal tragedy to share with strangers on the internet; give up my work once I can no longer reliably put words on a screen; manage with less money yet somehow pay someone else to walk my dog when I am too weak to do it . . . Does anyone know the password for my computer and, if not, how will they get into my email after I'm dead? I haven't stopped probing my neck all the while, my methodical fingers on autopilot, but I'm also now wondering what is involved in making a digital will.

When I finally snap out of this logistical reverie, my neck looks flushed and mottled in the mirror and the poking has finally woken up the few remaining nerves. They half-heartedly pull together an ache, but I can barely feel it. I haven't found anything definite and the panic ebbs ever so slightly. The subcutaneous ridges and hollows of scar tissue from previous operations give me some concern, but I know those of old. To know for sure if there is a real lump there, I need something better than just my clumsy fingers stabbing at the skin. I need to look from the inside. I need the knowledge and the equipment that turns opaque, ordinary flesh transparent, like glass, so that whatever is lurking within is exposed to the light. And to do that, I need help.

The first few times I experienced this panic at the office, I did what I thought I was supposed to do. I waited it out until the end of the working day somehow, and then I went to a walk-in clinic so that a nurse could prod my neck for a while. I tried to answer questions about what I thought I had felt, and condense my years-long medical history into a few brisk sentences, a sketch map of sorts for a newcomer to my personal medical labyrinth.

Each time the outcome was the same: the nurse couldn't feel anything so was unable to refer me for more tests, but also – given my history – wasn't prepared to give me the absolute, definite negative that would send me skipping home, my mind liberated from panic and free to worry about more mundane matters again, like what to pick up for dinner and whether there is really a wasps' nest growing in our attic. If I'm still worried, I am told for the umpteenth time, I should contact my previous doctors and make an appointment, but for now I need to stop bruising my neck or I'm going to inflame my old surgery wounds. I thank the nurse, button up my coat and go home. To have a consultation now, I'd have to take a day off work and several trains. It always ends the same way.

Whenever I receive this advice, I think about all the doctors I have seen in the past. About all the kind efforts to put my mind at ease, even though they cannot give me the guarantees that I want. About the symptoms that I have described, again and again, only to be told when tests for more serious conditions come back negative that I should lose a bit of weight or try to lower my stress levels. About how my mother once fainted and slid from her chair to the floor when a consultant delivered a life-altering diagnosis to her daughter. He just sat there and watched his words make her fall. I was seventeen and I hated him with a sudden searing passion that heated my body from the inside. Later, I used to daydream about making a miraculous recovery so I would never have to see him again.

After enough identical appointments like the one with the nurse about my neck, I stopped bothering to seek medical help when the shadow-tumour flickered into being. I could do my own examination, my own weighing up of probabilities. It was more efficient, I found, to surrender completely to the panic when it first surfaced, sneaking away to the office bathroom to know the worst before washing my face and returning to work. The sharp jabs of panic still hurt, but I know what I have to do to ride them out. Sometimes I can go from definitely dying to rude health inside half an hour.

This time, I'm almost there. The tears have dried up and a strange bubble of mirth bursts in my throat as I turn on the tap so I can splash my streaky face. My little chuckle echoes in the empty bathroom, the first sound I've made since I entered. All of the roaring was inside my head, as was the lump that I could feel but not see.

You are allowed to think it. I can hear you thinking it.

I am a hypochondriac. Or, at least, I worry that I am, which really amounts to the same thing.

The fear that there is something wrong with me, that I am sick, is always with me. I doubt that what I experience are physical sensations and I distrust my own interpretations of what I feel. Sometimes the anxiety is distant and muffled, like a radio playing in another room of the house, barely there. At other times, it is all I can hear.

Illness and the dread of it are entirely individual experiences – only I can have my sicknesses, real or not; only I can truly know how they feel – and, as such, hypochondria is very difficult to isolate or identify precisely. A self-help guide on the subject published by the UK's National Health Service tries to pin it down by including a transcript of common recurring thoughts that someone experiencing anxiety about their health might have; the second one on the list is 'I feel I am unwell.'

I have this thought almost every day.

It wasn't always this way. For the first sixteen years of my life, I was gloriously unaware of my own state of health. I experienced the usual cocktail of childhood maladies, from chicken pox to tonsillitis, but being ill was merely a temporary state that passed after a few days of rest and the ingestion of the right medicine. Once I was on my feet again, I never gave my sickbed a backwards glance. If I had thought about it, which I didn't, I would have said that I believed implicitly in the easy binaries of sickness and health: I was either well or I wasn't. To be healthy is to be oblivious, to enjoy the luxury of never having the degradation of the body intrude upon the mind. In the stories that I have told and retold myself about my sicknesses, these healthy years are a joyful blank, a silence filled with life.

The watershed in my understanding of myself, the before-and-after moment, came when I was seventeen and on the precipice of adulthood, cautiously looking over the edge at what my independent life might be like. I was applying to university, making new friends, getting serious about writing. Then a busy winter of feeling run-down culminated in me being diagnosed with Hodgkin's lymphoma, a relatively rare type of blood cancer. After months of treatment, I was given the all-clear and went off to university as planned. But then, during my first year at college, when I was eighteen, I found a lump in my neck that turned out to be a return of the cancer that was supposed to have been permanently purged from my body. I required more chemotherapy, a stem cell transplant and a weeks-long stay on an isolation ward – a sequence of progressively more invasive and dangerous treatments that ramped up as the persistent threat of this apparently curable cancer grew. Years of monitoring and testing followed before I was eventually declared cured at the age of twenty-two. The medical staff who had seen me through all of this waved me off with smiles, joking that they hoped never to see me again. Once I made it to five years after the end of the treatment, the likelihood of my getting cancer again had become about the same as for the rest of the population. There were no more annual check-ups, no more preventative medications, no more scans. My body and my life, they said, were cancer-free.

But I am not free.

Introduction

The People Made of Glass

Hypochondria is as slippery and elusive a term as the condition it tries to encompass. It dwells in contradictions: a perceived disease of the body that exists only in the mind. Within its shifting boundaries, the tangible and the intangible can change places and then change back again. It intersects with medicine but is the antithesis of the certainty that science attempts to provide. Hypochondria only has questions, never answers.

This condition resists definition, like oil sliding over the surface of water. This is not through want of effort: a vast and bewildering literature exists on this very subject. Hippocrates used the word in the fifth century BCE, and it has been a subject for study and discussion through every era since, but after centuries of work and acres of text, the question of what hypochondria is remains anything but settled. In 1909, Sigmund Freud told the Vienna Psychoanalytic Society that 'the position of hypochondria is still suspended in darkness', and more than a hundred years later it does not feel as if there is much more light on the subject. Even in the most widely used and up-to-date clinical literature, its definition is still shifting and changing. For instance, for the latest edition of the *Diagnostic and Statistical Manual* (*DSM-5*), which was published in 2013 by the American Psychiatric Association and is often referred to as 'the bible of psychiatry', the diagnosis of hypochondria was entirely recategorised into two separate entities: somatic symptom disorder and illness anxiety disorder. Both describe patients with 'extensive worries about health', but the former features so-called somatic or physical symptoms the patient feels in their body which medicine cannot detect or explain, whereas the latter is focused solely on 'preoccupation with having or acquiring a serious illness' and 'excessive health-related behaviours'.

Reading the *DSM-5* is a confusing experience. The first time is comforting, even exciting. Here I am, inscribed with supreme authority in the pages of this highly influential text that informs the diagnostic efforts of medical experts everywhere. The list of likely symptoms matches up with me. I am 'easily alarmed about personal health status' and I have been like this for more than six months, with the specific illness that I fear shifting often. Under illness anxiety disorder, two 'types' are listed and I am definitely of the 'care seeking' rather than 'care avoidant' type, although I am aware of fellow sufferers who have reacted to similar circumstances to mine in the opposite way, refusing to seek medical attention at all in case bad news is delivered.

On subsequent readings, though, the *DSM-5* loses its lustre of certainty. It begins to seem less like a dictionary and more like an extensive exercise in obfuscation. Although there is plenty that I recognise in these pages, I don't seem to fit consistently into either of the two successor disorders to hypochondria: I exhibit some of the aspects of both, some of the time. To be diagnosed with illness anxiety disorder rather than somatic symptom disorder, my somatic symptoms must be 'only mild in intensity', but there is no assistance offered with what is mild and what is not. The book contains too many over-lapping possibilities to offer clarity. Conditions like obsessive compulsive disorder, body dysmorphic disorder, some eating disorders and generalised anxiety disorder are considered closely related, and the boundaries between these conditions and hypochondria are blurred.

Plenty of experts in this field are just as sceptical about the *DSM-5*'s latest attempt to define hypochondria. The authors of one study, looking for evidence among a cohort of real patients that the new criteria helped to alleviate their anxieties and symptoms, concluded that replacing the single condition of hypochondria with these two new disorders was unhelpful or, in the devastating yet impersonal language of medical research, it 'appears rather contradictory and incompatible with former diagnostic concepts and current cognitive behavioural models of hypochondriasis and health anxiety'. This mirrors my own experience with the *DSM-5*: at a quick glance, it seems to have finally sliced through the knotty, ancient problem of hypochon-dria, but upon closer inspection, it has merely added another layer of tangles.

Even selecting our vocabulary for this fear is fraught with difficulty. I once used the word 'hypochondria' during a con-sultation with a doctor, only to have him chuckle and pull a brand new medical dictionary off the shelf to show me that the term had now been deemed 'obsolete'. This is the word that I know, that responds when I reach for something to name the collection of fears and feelings that exists inside me, but it is far from a settled designation.

We tend to think of hypochondria as shorthand for an illness that's all in your head, but the word we use today was born of a

medieval term for an area of the abdomen. Theorists traditionally divided the body below the breastbone into nine distinct
areas, a three by three square that makes a neat, flat grid from
the three-dimensional curves of the human torso. The squares
on the top left and top right are known as the two hypochondriac regions, or the 'hypochondrium', with one square
corresponding to the liver and the other to the spleen and
parts of the stomach. For more than a thousand years, during
which time the dissection of human bodies was extremely rare,
this way of mapping and naming the abdomen was accepted
unchallenged by the medical scholars and practitioners of
Europe, North Africa and the Middle East.

The parts that make up the word 'hypochondria' are much
older though. In the Greek of Hippocrates and his contemporaries, *hupo* meant 'under' and *khondros* denoted the cartilage
of the sternum. With these two parts combined, almost like
the coordinates of a map reference, this word was adopted
into Latin and then arrived in English in the fifteenth century. For many centuries, hypochondria, the plural form of
the word referring to the two mirrored sections of the torso,
was merely a geographical term used to narrow down where
a swelling or pain was located rather than a condition in its
own right. But then something changed: by the seventeenth
century it had come to denote the mysterious and melancholy
condition thought to result from an imbalance of black bile
and vapours in the organs of these regions. Gradually, the
physical specificity of the word faded away and any illness
without a detectable cause began to be referred to as 'hypochondria', until it arrived at today's definition of 'the persistent
and unwarranted belief or fear that one has a serious illness'.
Without changing a syllable, it has come down to us with a new
meaning that still contains the old description of these internal

organs. The word is at once visceral and figurative, just like the condition that it describes.

I only began to doubt my own comfort with this term once I became better acquainted with the modern medical debate around it. For most of the twentieth century, the academic work on this subject preferred *hypochondriasis*, which has the benefit of being a complicated, long word that lends an air of authority to a field that has few certainties about it. The addition of the *-asis* suffix is an archaic trick that arrived in English from Greek via Latin, having long been used as a way of transforming ordinary nouns into medical conditions. Thus, 'elephant' became *elephantiasis*, a condition that causes the skin to roughen and crack until it resembles an elephant's hide, and 'arsenic' became *arseniasis*, denoting the symptoms arising from chronic arsenic poisoning. Adding *-asis* to words is part of how medical expertise is underpinned by language.

It is unsurprising, then, that *hypochondriasis* was the label used in the *DSM-IV*, published in 1994. It was a subheading under the general umbrella of 'somataform disorders' – a catch-all term for conditions which include 'the presence of physical symptoms that suggest a general medical condition and are not fully explained by a general medical condition'. This desig-nation had its dissenters, though. A boldly titled 2004 study proposing 'a new, empirically established hypochondriasis diag-nosis' suggested dropping 'the stigmatising hypochondriasis label' in favour of 'health anxiety', although the authors weren't even completely confident about that. In the next few lines, they proposed 'valetudin disorder' instead, a relatively recent coinage from 1988 that comes from the Greek word *valetudo*, meaning 'state of health'. Valetudo was also what the Romans called Hygieia, the Greek goddess of health, cleanliness and hygiene. It's a neat way of tying up several loose ends and highlighting the strong connections contemporary medicine still has with the ancient world, but 'valetudin disorder' as a name has not caught on at all. I have never seen it anywhere other than in this paper, although I am fond of the eighteenth-century word 'valetudinarian' to designate 'a person of a weak or sickly constitution'. It sounds so illustrious, somehow.

The further I travel into this convoluted maze of medical jargon and historical etymology, the more it becomes clear that names have enormous power here. In the last two decades, the point of contention has shifted somewhat: scholars are no longer arguing only about what hypochondria *is*, but about what words they should use while they have that argument. In a more empathetic, less judgemental era of medicine, people in this field feel a responsibility to acknowledge and even reverse the harm done by the medical language of the past. The simple act of speaking these words comes with centuries of baggage associated with who is believed when they speak of their pain, and who is not. Marginalised people – be they women, those who aren't white, the disabled, the poor or the less educated – have long been considered by those in authority to be less reliable witnesses to their own symptoms and sensations. Terms like 'somatoform disorder' should be abolished, it is argued, because patients don't like the doubt inherent in the phrase. The unnecessary inclusion of *somato-*, a prefix meaning 'bodily', suggests that their symptoms are merely a delusional manifestation of a mental disorder and thus not considered genuine, tangible or treatable by doctors. 'The disorders mainly characterised by medically unexplained physical symptoms *are real*,' one expert earnestly concludes, as if an italic font can make up for past derision. Something pings in my head when I read this – *are mental disorders not also real?* In my experience, medical professionals today tend to default to the term 'health

anxiety', which seems to blend in well with the current practical vocabulary of mental health, while in conversation most
people still say hypochondria, blissfully unaware of the millennia of turmoil that follow the word like the tail of a comet.

I like the word 'hypochondria'. I cannot abandon it. It feels
rooted in a history and a tradition that connects sufferers
stretching back over 2,000 years. It offers companionship while
in the grip of a fear that can be completely isolating. It provides
edges to a feeling of uncertainty that, in bad moments, can feel
like it stretches on forever. At times, it can even offer relief: if
this is 'just hypochondria', my health is safe from other threats,
for now. A name is a powerful spell. Of all the terms I have
encountered in my strange voyage through the backstory of
this condition, it is the one most instantly recognisable to most
people, and thus the one that I will use most often in this book.
I deliberately use it imprecisely, allowing the term to encompass everything from acute and incapacitating delusions to the
low-level yet persistent anxiety that gnaws at many of us in the
course of everyday life. To have meaning, the word must be as
indistinct and flexible as the condition it denotes.

In part, I do this because I would like to claim this word
for myself. But, according to some experts, the absolutely
classic definition of hypochondria does not apply to me. My
fears about my health are persistent and at times intrusive, but
they are not necessarily unwarranted. I have been diagnosed
with cancer once already and had it recur to the surprise of the
experts treating me. Perhaps it is not unreasonable or irrational,
then, to worry that either that same cancer or the effects of
the powerfully harmful treatments I received for it could still
be lingering in my body causing mischief. I find myself dissatisfied with this rationale, though. While it is undoubtedly

true that some of my health-related behaviours – the checking for lumps in places where they have previously been excised, for instance – are directly related to my medical history, what might once have been a proportionate level of anxiety has long since swelled into something all of its own. My status as a former cancer patient is both an enormous privilege and a perpetual curse: it means that I survived and that my symptoms are always investigated thoroughly, but it also means that I have long been encouraged by doctors to pay close attention to how I feel in case I can pick up an early warning sign of a recurrence or a side effect. This habit of constant scanning is also a mixed blessing. It once caught a new tumour in good time, but it also means that I notice changes in how my body feels that bear no resemblance to anything involved in Hodgkin's lymphoma. It is the reason I become convinced that I have some entirely separate and new but life-threatening condition, even when doctors can find no evidence to support my concerns or links to my previous conditions. It feels at times like having cancer for real was the training I went through so that I could have a dozen other illnesses in my imagination. I am now very *good* at being unwell. I've had a lot of practice.

The longer I have lived with this, the more I have become convinced that diagnosable illness and hypochondria can coexist. One is not the antithesis of the other. They are intimate companions, and in someone with my history and tendencies, they are forever pushing each other to new heights. The perfectly healthy person with no detectable ailments who nonetheless lives with the constant belief that they are sick is a rarity, more common in theory than in life. Most people have some legitimate concern about at least one aspect of their health, whether it is a prior condition, a family history or an environmental factor. Hypochondria creeps in when this justifiable anxiety expands well beyond the boundaries of the verifiable health concern; when someone with a chronic back injury becomes convinced that they have mouth cancer, say. Even those who society holds up as exemplars of athleticism can fall prey to these patterns of thought; a very fit friend who suffered a sports injury years ago is still constantly monitoring and treading carefully on a right foot that the experts say is now as sound as the left. The manifold difficulties of this relationship between illness real and imagined lie in drawing those boundaries. Who gets to decide what is reasonable fear and what is unreasonable? Medicine is always evolving and improving too; it is now possible to test for conditions that were previously undetectable. The firm, logical basis upon which today's evidence-based diagnoses stand is in fact shifting, ever so slightly, every time new research is undertaken and new results are published. Nothing is certain for ever. Everyone has their niggling doubts, that internal voice that says *what if?* The hypochondriacs are just listening out for it that much more keenly.

Everything about my situation – the hypochondriac cancer survivor – feels quixotic and a bit silly, as if some higher being finds the absurdity of my juxtapositions amusing. It took being cured of a life-threatening illness for me to become fixated on the idea that I might be sick. Now, health for me is mostly the absence of illness, never a state to be appreciated for its own sake. My anxiety is rooted in the idea that disease could be lurking undetected, ready to consume me at any time. After all, my fears have not always been groundless. It's just that at the moment, the scans say there is nothing there. The symptoms haunt the edges of my perception, always tugging at my attention. I feel like my own unreliable narrator, always delivering only a partial account of how I feel, never quite able to make others understand. Am I a hypochondriac, or am I just a responsible patient? I can't ever ignore what I feel, because what if, this time, I am right and the thing that almost felled me before is back again?

Although I wish I could believe that all my fears were imaginary, the whole notion of hypochondria feels at times like a medical hoax. Why am I simultaneously drawn to and suspicious of this label? The more I have studied the history of the condition, the more this doubt of mine feels, ironically, like yet another symptom of hypochondria itself. I'm so consumed by doubt about my body's ability to stay healthy and by my mind's turmoil that I'm not even willing to award myself this, the broadest and most vague of diagnoses. This is partly because hypochondria is a label that will not necessarily secure me understanding and compassion from others – if anything, the reverse, since there is still substantial stigma attached to experiencing unconfirmed or imaginary illnesses. For some, their presence hints at a mind that might be delusional, even unstable. Some of you reading this now, whether friend, acquaintance or stranger, will probably think less of me in some private, secret way for sharing this part of myself. I used to worry about that, but now I just think: I am glad you don't know what it is like.

While I have sometimes found it hard to talk about my experiences to people I know, I have had a long-running conversation with the hypochondriacs of centuries past who committed their fears to paper. Often they do not show themselves immediately. This is one of the many strange things about this condition and the word that describes it: everybody knows what it means and – if my experiences while writing this book are at all typical – knows somebody who suffers from it, but it is rarely used in official documents or proclamations. It is extremely unusual to find an obituary that mentions it, for instance, even if it was a major feature of the deceased's life. It is too inconclusive, too shameful, too silly to mention. To find my hypochondriac fellow travellers, then, I had to dig a little deeper, into memoirs, letters and autobiographies. This inevitably narrows the field: only those notable enough to be written about, or sufficiently talented and appreciated that their writing has been preserved, are available for investigation.

Nevertheless, I have built teetering piles of hypochondriacal lives. Robert Burton, Caspar Barlaeus, Constantijn Huygens, John Donne, Blaise Pascal, Elizabeth Barrett Browning, Marcel Proust, Hans Christian Andersen, Tennessee Williams, Howard Hughes, Alice James, Glenn Gould, James Madison – the list is extensive and broad, encompassing poets, presidents, musicians, clerics and many others. For all of them, their hypochondriacal impulses coexisted with diagnosed and treated conditions, often to the extent that it can be difficult for us, as it surely was for them, to tell where that boundary between fictional and real illness is. This I find reassuring: if my pre-existing conditions mean I don't fit the true definition of a hypochondriac, then I am in good company. Proust, for instance, suffered from early childhood with severe hay fever and allergies that the family doctor considered real enough to treat multiple times with a painful nasal cauterising procedure, but when the young Marcel continued to struggle with terrible attacks of breathlessness even after this supposed 'cure' had been administered, those around him began to wonder if all of his symptoms were physical in origin. His father, a prominent epidemiologist and noted expert on cholera, especially seems to have had his doubts. Difficulty breathing was strongly associated with hysteria and so-called nervous disorders in the late nineteenth century, and Adrien Proust suspected that his son's symptoms arose from some inherent sensitivity of character, rather than actual disease. When Marcel was twenty-eight, he wrote to his mother from the spa town of Évian-les-Bains about how his friends had mocked him because he had declined to travel there by car and had instead gone by train on his own, for fear that the rush of cold air outside would bring on an asthma attack:

> Constantine said I just imagined that cold air was bad for me, because Papa told everyone that my asthma was purely imaginary. I know only too well when I awake here in the morning that it is quite real.

Illness is so individual and becomes such a large part of our identity that we unconsciously ascribe personality traits to it – for ourselves and for those around us. Why not also apply them to the illnesses of those who have gone before? When my undetectable symptoms are making it difficult for me to put my mind to anything else, I silently berate myself for being lazy and selfish, as if there is something inherent about my character that causes these disruptive sensations, that they come from within rather than without. Over time, Proust became the delicate and sensitive person that his father feared he already was. He developed elaborate rituals for his household to follow that were intended to protect him from dust, pollen and smells, and he rarely risked going outside, where an attack might take him unawares. When he did travel, he did his best to replicate his rarefied home environment. Eventually, his fears led to behaviours that ultimately made his health worse: terrified of the smoke from fires, he existed in largely unheated rooms, and fearing the effect of cooking smells, he ate less and less. The drugs he took to mitigate his symptoms also weakened him to the point where he contracted secondary infections like influenza. In a case like this, the original sickness, the fear of its recurrence, the steps taken to treat it and the personality of the patient all meld into one living, coughing, suffering being. There is no point wondering if I, or Proust, or any of these other hypochondriacs would have been different had they never been ill in the first place: there is no alternative, healthy, existence.

The author John Green once described his mind and his body as 'two old friends who have drifted apart but are still required by circumstance to spend all their time together', and I recognised what he meant immediately. That awkwardly forced companionship while wishing the other was far, far away accurately describes the disjointed way I have envisioned myself for a very long time. In yoga classes or meditation sessions when the leader says something like 'think yourself into your body for a moment and feel its connection to the earth', a rebellious part of me always silently responds: *why would I want to do that?* The separation I maintain between mind and body keeps me safe from feeling and endlessly interpreting every single twinge and ache. If I have to inhabit a fragile meat vessel that could disintegrate at any moment, at least don't make me think about it all the time.

Hypochondria puts a magnifying glass to the ancient problem of mind versus body. Philosophers from every culture have for millennia been debating the exact site of consciousness in the human self, and whether the generation of thought is a physical process similar to, say, sneezing, or something else entirely. So much rides on this: the nature of the soul, what happens to us after death, the very essence of creativity and existence. Some have argued for a separation, the primacy of mind over body or body over mind, while others prefer to think of them as two sides of one whole. In Buddhism, the mind is a sixth sense that operates just like sight or sound or touch, which raises interesting possibilities for being able to separate self, thought and soul. More recently, the interconnectedness of mind and body has been increasingly underpinned by medical discovery. Mindset and stress can have a huge impact on physical sensation, while the composition of microbes in the gut seems to be able to exert a powerful influence over the brain. Against the backdrop of all this, we have hypochondria, a condition once thought to inhabit the body that has gradually become a problem of the mind, but which also causes physical symptoms that seem to be only mental in origin – or at least cannot be pinned to a so-called organic cause by existing tests. The word 'real' is used a lot in this arena, in the sense that only physical symptoms verified externally are truly happening, and something that is felt 'only in the head' is therefore unreal.

Hypochondriacs are perhaps more aware than other people of this fundamental divide between body and mind. Proust's narrator in *The Guermantes Way* argues that it is only in the experience of being sick that we are forced to confront that otherness, the alien horror of our corporeality:

> It is in sickness that we are compelled to recognise that we do not live alone but are chained to a being from a different realm, from whom we are worlds apart, who has no knowledge of us and by whom it is impossible to make ourselves understood: our body.

Hypochondriacs may be more aware of what happens in the body, but they are also more reluctant to feel it. We are hypervigilant to even the slightest change because it could indicate that something sinister is happening, but at the same time wary of seeking help for something that is just going to be branded, shamefully, 'not real' – or worse, seeking help and

discovering that it *is* real. Hence the deliberate distance maintained between mind and body, even while being constantly
aware of its nuances. I need to know so that I can decide when
it is time to act. I have become so used to the constant, intensive monitoring of my body that I feel a jolt of shock every time
I realise that most healthy people are lucky enough to go year
to year with very minimal contact with their doctor. What my
husband affectionately refers to as 'my ailments' are a perpetual presence in my life; I am rarely not being investigated for
something. If the full range of my everyday mental preoccupations were to be expressed as a pie chart, the segment labelled
'health' would occupy about a third of the whole, waxing as I
find new, alarming symptoms and waning when others recede.
During the worst times, the health slice grows inexorably and
consumes everything else, until all I have in my head is the
throbbing monotony of being unable to think about anything
other than whether I am teetering on the brink of an unpleasant
discovery. This is, as I constantly berate myself, a giant waste
of time and energy. And yet I cannot stop.

   While there is comfort to be found in knowing that others,
like Proust, have shared my preoccupations, I am also aware
that my experience of my body and my knowledge of all the
things that could go wrong with it are shaped by the era in
which I live. The history of hypochondria and that of medicine are permanently interwoven, like the ivy and the tree
around which it is entwined, forever growing together. At every
advance, every new medical discovery, hypochondria has taken
a step forward too. Our fears keep pace with our knowledge.
As science reveals more of the workings of our bodies, making
them ever more transparent to us, we find new and fertile
ground for fear.

                              *

In the second century CE, the Greek physician Galen of Pergamon noted the existence of a peculiar condition, seemingly all in the patient's mind but felt in the body: 'Fears always accompany melancholic people, but they do not always get the same kind of unnatural imaginations. For instance, the one thinks that he is a piece of pottery so that he avoids those who approach him in order not to be broken.' There are references to this phenomenon in other physicians' accounts too, along with attempts to rationalise it into the medicine of the time. Rufus of Ephesus, another second-century physician and medical writer, suggests that patients of a cold, dry disposition are more likely to fall prey to the idea that they are made of a brittle clay, and the notion is later picked up enthusiastically by Aëtius of Amida, a Byzantine physician of the fifth and sixth centuries. He noted that, along with believing that one had been transformed into a chicken or being mortally afraid that the sky was about to fall, this transformation into pottery remained in the first rank of unexplained delusions a few centuries after Galen's initial identification.

Then in the late fourteenth century, this preoccupation with earthenware abruptly changed. The patients of this era shared many of the same anxieties as their pottery-fixated antecedents, feeling fragile, brittle and extremely smashable, but they no longer believed their flesh had been transformed into baked clay, but that it had become a new material: glass. Although humans had been working with glass in various ways for thousands of years, it wasn't until the method known as the crown glass process was perfected in late-thirteenth-century Venice that glass-making became a recognisable and widespread trade in Europe. As more people grew familiar with the process and its products, those inclined towards delusions of fragility and impermanence were drawn to the symbolic potential of glass.

This delusion is not hypochondria in the strictest sense, although it is a fitting touchstone for the complex knot of emotions and sensations that we now associate with the word. What these people believed afflicted them was not a recognisable illness but a wholesale bodily transformation into a material utterly unlike human flesh. Usually classified as sufferers from mania or melancholy, these 'glass people' took different forms. Some believed that they had assumed the form of a particular glass object, such as an oil lamp or a jar, while in rare cases, the entire substance of the person was transformed into glass. Individual body parts could be afflicted too, while the rest of the body remained unaffected. Glass limbs were reported, but glass hearts and heads were far more common. The places where the mind and body meet, where it feels like the self resides, seemed to be most susceptible. One, possibly exaggerated, report from the early seventeenth century by a French royal physician concerned a Parisian glassmaker who suffered from a form of the delusion focused on the buttocks. He supposedly went around with a small cushion fastened to his behind at all times, in case it broke when he sat down. He was apparently cured by a doctor who beat him severely until he accepted that it was flesh which hurt so badly and that he hadn't broken. This story recurs across multiple places and sources – it is in a sixteenth-century treatise by a Dutch physician, then in an early-seventeenth-century English cleric's book about the four humours, and in an allegorical play from 1607 titled *Lingua, or the Combat of the Tongue*, in which a character declares 'I am an Urinal I dare not stirre, / For fear of cracking in the Bottome.' I think part of the reason that this particular instance recurs so much is because it is both funny and absurd, indicating that hypochondria is often treated as ridiculous or a joke 'illness' which requires those inverted commas.

The first person who believed themselves to be entirely made of glass was the French King Charles VI (or at least as far as we know; the delusions of less important people are not so well documented). In 1392, during a military campaign in the north-west of his kingdom, the twenty-four-year-old Charles was gripped by a mania and, according to those around him, suddenly transformed into a completely different person. He started talking nonsense, would not respond to reason and tried to attack his own soldiers. His courtiers restrained him and took him back to Paris, where his ravings coalesced around a specific fear. He could not bear to be touched, he said, because he was made of glass and could shatter on contact. He had his clothing reinforced with iron rods and always moved with caution because a collision could break him apart. His condition led to a regency battle and then a civil war between armies led by his brothers and his wife. In a sense, the French state shattered because its monarch believed he was made of glass.

The glass delusion was still thriving in the seventeenth century when Cervantes published his 1613 novella *El licenciado Vidriera*, or *The Glass Graduate*. It follows the fortunes of one Tomás Rodaja, a law student poisoned by a suitor with an aphrodisiac potion. He hovers between life and death for months, but his doctors eventually manage to cure his physical symptoms. His recovery is only partial, though, because his mind is afflicted by 'the strangest madness that was ever heard of among the many kinds by which humanity has been assailed'.

Tomás, like Charles VI, believes himself to be entirely made of glass from head to foot. He becomes terrified that the slightest touch will cause him to break into pieces. His friends and doctors try to appeal to his sense of reason – he was a lawyer, after all – and prove that he will not shatter by forcibly embracing him. Tomás merely faints from terror and has no memory of the experiments when he wakes hours later. He asks that anyone speaking to him stands a good way off, just in case, and he takes to sleeping in the open air during summer to avoid any nocturnal collisions. In winter, he buries himself in straw up to the throat every night as if he is a precious vessel being packed away for a journey. The year after this story was published, a royal physician recorded that an unnamed French prince had adopted the same tactic, refusing to leave his straw bed for fear of breakage. In that case, a cure was effected by setting fire to the locked room in which he languished – the glass man turned back to flesh in time to hammer on the door and save himself.

In Cervantes' story there is an interesting twist on the inherent folly of Tomás's delusion, as he finds that because he is now composed of 'a substance of more delicate subtlety', he is more sensitive to the nature of the world and to the problems of others. He becomes sought after for his wise counsel, and even 'the most learned professors of medicine and philosophy' are astonished that a man operating under such a fundamental delusion about the nature of his own body can be so astute.

The preoccupation with glass endured for as long as the material was considered novel and special, peaking in the late seventeenth century and then diminishing as glass became commonplace – something that we barely notice. It hasn't vanished entirely, though. A case of full-blown glass delusion was recorded in the Netherlands as recently as 1964. This final glass man had different worries from his predecessors. Reflecting the way that glass had become much stronger, less breakable and more reliable over the centuries, this patient was not concerned that he would break, but rather that he was completely transparent and thus invisible. He explained his condition by directing his doctor's attention to a nearby window, then saying: 'That's me. I'm there, and I'm not there. Like the glass in the window.'

What all these glass people had in common was a dual obsession with their fragility and transparency. They felt both highly breakable and completely exposed. In its modern incarnation, the hypochondriac idea of a body made of glass is not only a symptom of anxiety, it also holds out the possibility of a cure. Through scans and blood tests, biopsies and surgery, X-rays and genome analysis, the body is being rendered increasingly transparent to medical and scientific knowledge. If we can *see* that all is well, or if we can pinpoint the exact nature of what is wrong, perhaps our bigger fears will disappear. And yet, with this transparency comes an awareness of the million minute things that need to function well for us to be healthy and the ease with which any of them could fail. Until advanced imaging techniques became widely available, very few people feared that their intermittent headaches and flashing vision were the result of hidden brain tumours. Instead, they were preoccupied by whatever the condition *du jour* was: plague, fever, consumption, AIDS. The impulse to be afraid of our bodies and what they can do remains, but the precise form that this takes has changed over time. Hypochondria is not tied to any one condition or type of disease, but rather to the essence of the doubt itself. Wherever medicine reaches the extent of its powers, there lies hesitation, suspicion and confusion. And those are the raw materials from which hypochondria is formed.

When early modern scholars recorded instances of the glass delusion, they were writing literally. There is no indication that the patients they observed were speaking metaphorically: when sufferers said 'I think I am made of glass', they meant that it felt as if some or all of their flesh had somehow taken on the properties associated with that material: hardness, transparency, fragility. But long after physical instances of the delusion had dwindled, the concept of a glass body has lingered in the collective imagination. In Spanish, the phrase *licenciado vidriera* is an idiom meaning an excessively delicate and shy person, and in English we use the word 'fragile' to describe a state of less than robust health, either mental or physical, without meaning that the person will literally shatter upon contact. The brittle nature of glass has become part of how we describe ourselves, even if Charles VI with his reinforced clothing has receded into the realm of absurdity.

The more I have learned about the glass people of centuries past, the more I have become convinced that their affliction is the perfect analogue for beginning to understand an ancient condition that remakes itself anew for every age. Hypochondria exists at the intersection of those feelings of fragility and transparency experienced by the glass people. We are breakable. We are vulnerable. We are baffling. We are ungovernable. We are misunderstood, ridiculed, ignored.

When I experience an episode of severe anxiety about my health, I become an unreliable narrator of my own body. The fear makes me partial; I only pay attention to what fits my belief that I am sick. Lumps that nobody else can feel are real to me, and hair comes out in my hands for no reason that anybody can find. There must be an underlying cause that connects it all, I reason, and my brain scrabbles uselessly against the edifice of this disease that only I can sense. That common, bracing injunction that 'you probably imagined it' can feel a lot like those friends of Tomás Rodaja attempting to prove to him that he was not made of glass by trying to break him with their embraces. A kindness that crushes.

In one version of the glass delusion, sufferers believed not that their flesh had been transformed into glass, but that they were irrevocably trapped inside such a vessel. James Howell, an agent for an English glass factory, wrote in a letter to his brother from Venice dated 1 June 1621 that he had learned of a man there who believed himself to be held inside a glass urinal. Howell's erudite comment was 'surely he deserved to be piss'd in the Mouth'. It was long before I learned of the glass delusion that I started having my own daydreams of bodies in glass vessels. Many years prior to cancer making my body a strange and painful place to be, I felt disjointed and malcoordinated, lacking the physical grace and speed that I observed in those around me. My mind moved at a pace I felt proud of, but my body was always dragging behind: too slow, the wrong shape, either shivering or burning. How much better life would be, I would muse, if I could be just a mind, a brain in a jar. Later, this became a mental defence mechanism to the impositions of illness and anxiety: if I can keep what feels like my self separate from the treacherous battleground of lumps and scars, then the essential part of me is safe.

Illness is a story we tell about ourselves. The narrative is the connective tissue that joins together the symptoms and perceptions and makes sense of them. It's how impenetrable concepts like death and life become something that can be incorporated comfortably into day-to-day existence. A serious illness is much easier to cope with if it can be slotted into a familiar structure with a beginning, middle and end. It's also why metaphors of battle or struggle are so popular for describing sickness. It draws the line between them and us, good and evil. To say that someone 'lost their struggle with cancer' is to impart meaning to their death. The mind shies away from senseless tragedy. We want everything to have happened for a reason, even if it didn't.

This urge towards narrative forms a vital part of hypochondria too, as the sufferer tries to weave their disparate sensations into the pattern of a recognisable condition as a way of staving off the yawning blackness of the unknown. According to the novelist Benjamin Hale, humans 'are meaning makers ... We make meanings because meaninglessness terrifies us above all things.' This instinct is in part why hypochondria is so difficult to isolate and treat. It is deeply connected to other aspects of the psyche, such as conditions like depression, or personality traits like a propensity for worry.

In my desperation to find a rationale for my own episodes of anxiety about my health over the years, I have looked for a pattern in how and when they occur. I've found that although it is possible for an imaginary lump to burst into being on an otherwise good day, I am much more likely to get pulled into my familiar maelstrom of horrors if I am already at a low ebb emotionally. Negative thoughts seem to flow seamlessly into those about my health: perhaps I am feeling like a professional failure because of a recent rejection, so my body must be failing me too. As much as I think I would like a dispassionate diagnosis of some verifiable condition, I also recognise that what ails me is unlikely to show up in any medical textbook because it is me. Only I have my feelings, and only I have my hypochondria.

The first time a doctor meets a new patient, they take a 'history'. This is an account of the illness from the perspective of the body hosting it, but because we are people rather than just a jumble of symptoms, it will inevitably include other things. Like details about environment, personality, family, bias, fear and joy. This is the stuff that the MRI machine cannot see: the image of the patient only visible to themselves. The history obtained by the doctor will be partial and might not make sense all the time. Some of it will not seem relevant at the time when it is first spoken aloud. It will be contradicted, expanded and modified by the results of future tests, scans and examinations.

It is the product of a particular moment and meeting; if I were not the patient, and this were not my doctor, the history would read completely differently. Despite all of these caveats, the history is an attempt, a vitally important one, to make something out of nothing. To find meaning where before there was none.

Being able to take the malleable, changeable, contradictory properties of a medical history and apply them to an entire condition rather than a person is what first drew me to writing about hypochondria. This is a condition that breathes and changes; this kind of living biography feels like the best way to capture it. This version of the tale can only be told by me, here and now, and is shaped by this moment in time as well as everything that has gone before. That is why this book is *a* history of hypochondria, not *the* history. Rather than endeavour to create some grisly chimera formed out of the dictionary and encyclopaedia, I am seeking clarity over comprehensiveness. I am pulling on the fragile thread of our doubt as it weaves through every age of medical progress, stitching together the mind and the body, and connecting the visceral days of black bile in the spleen and therapeutic bleedings to the 3 a.m. 'should this hurt?' Google searches.

Gently, tenderly, I will hold the body made of glass to the light and watch it shine.

I

The Origins of the Ancient Malady

Hypochondria has been called 'the ancient malady' and for good reason. For as long as humans have had an understanding of health, there has been anxiety about it, and it has resisted explanation or understanding. It is in part because the condition is so impervious to comprehension or cure that it has endured; the precise nature of hypochondria in any given time depends so much on the context of each moment in which it manifests. There is a continuity in its transformation from age to age: a patient living on a small Greek island in the fifth century BCE could use the word and be understood by their doctor, just as I can today, albeit we would be referring to very different sensations and ailments. Medicine is a field so defined by improvement and progress, ever eager to evolve, to supersede old theories with newer, better ones. This point of connection between past and present – a survival of something old, still experienced anew – feels consequential. It tells us something about the unaltering essence of what it is to be alive, sick and afraid. In this way, hypochondria is a mirror: it reflects the doubts of each new era back to us, an act of doubling that allows us to catch a glimpse of the soft, fearful underbelly that mostly stays out of sight when we peruse the history of medicine.

The doubt inherent in medicine, and upon which hypochondria feeds, has been present in every time, at every sickbed and clinical consultation, in every apothecary shop and laboratory. It was there when Byzantine physicians in the sixth century BCE were trying to drain excess phlegm from their patients in an attempt to cure epilepsy, and it is there now as a cancer researcher painstakingly tests an experimental new treatment on clusters of cells while observing them through a powerful microscope. There is a symmetry to this, to how we behave in the presence of a threat to our health, whether it is ultimately proved to be real or imagined. Disease and the fear of disease: we flip between the alternatives unceasingly – *I'm sure, I'm not sure.* The path between these two extremes is clustered with cliché, a reassuring indication of how many have passed this way before. Better to be safe than sorry. If only I had known. I never felt a thing.

Even before there was a word for it, the foundations were being laid for hypochondria deep in the human psyche. It is, in fact, built into the complex web of adaptations and traits that enabled our evolution and survival. Behavioural researchers make a compelling case that developing the ability to monitor health and identify potential threats to it were essential evolutionary steps for early humans, and that excessive anxiety about health grew out of this crucial skill.

From the very beginning, there was a fundamental contradiction at the heart of our existence: the same close social contact that enabled the ultimate goal of living beings, reproduction, also intensified the risk of dying without offspring via violence or disease. Studies at the genetic level have shown how infectious diseases were one of the main causes of death in human communities 100,000 years ago. That same research has revealed how much genetic adaptation was driven by the microbes, viruses and parasites with which these early humans came into contact – those who did not succumb to a potentially fatal disease were forever altered by the encounter, and when these mutations aided survival, they were passed on. Indeed, some genetic differences between human populations in different areas of the world can be traced back to variations in the profile of infectious diseases encountered in the local environment.

Physiological responses – what we commonly refer to as the immune system – were and are a crucial line of defence against disease. The ability of the body to detect and resist a dangerous pathogen is, of course, the difference between survival and death. But in these early days of human adaptation and selection, another form of protection began to take shape, one that could prevent the threat from ever entering the body at all. This behavioural immune system was formed from signals and responses that enabled the brain to recognise possible sources of infection and prompt the individual to avoid contact with them altogether. Evading illness, so that the body never had to deploy a physiological immune response, played a key role in survival, limiting the risk of infection and increasing the chance of survival if infected. The development of disgust, especially towards potential sources of infection such as dirt, rotten food and carriers of disease, was a vital component of this form of self-protection – it was a way of parsing the disparate clues to potential harm and collecting them together under a single emotional response. Disgust even played a role in helping early humans determine which creatures to fear; studies have shown a positive correlation between disease avoidance, the food rejection aspect of disgust, and common fears of specific animals. Recognising the signs of sickness in other individuals and animals and taking action to avoid them became an instinctive part of maintaining health.

The logic for some of this behaviour is very apparent: don't eat food that is emitting a rotten smell, don't approach or touch the individual with the open weeping sores and the hacking cough. And this isn't just in our past. Traces of this relationship are still evident in our makeup today. A common symptom both during early pregnancy and just before menstruation is a heightened sense of smell, caused by raised hormone levels, which can make even the most previously innocuous food or fragrance seem repulsive. The endocrine system is an intrinsic part of this behavioural immune system, and elevating a woman's disgust level at these crucial moments in her reproductive journey is a way of the body taking extra precautions to ensure the survival of the next generation. But these detection abilities, rooted in what is coded as 'disgusting', go much further than the obvious connection between bad smells and bad food. Much more subtle sensory clues, such as a slight swelling to the face or a marginally different kind of body odour, can indicate the presence of a disease long before the more overt signs become evident. Once this behavioural immune system is operating, the observer might not even be conscious that something smells off, so to speak, but they will experience an urge to give the newcomer a wide berth.

Fascinatingly, humans still do this without even being aware of the mechanisms involved. A study carried out in 2021 at the University of California tested this by putting participants in an MRI machine while they looked at photographs of different faces and answered questions about which they found most likeable. Some of the people in the pictures had been injected with a mild bacterial infection and others had received only a placebo. The photos of the infected people were rated as less likeable, and the least liked faces were those experiencing the greatest inflammatory response to the injected toxin – a clear demonstration of the unconscious ability to sort sickness from health, even with limited sensory input. Researchers also observed a noticeable increase in activity in the ventromedial prefrontal cortex (vmPFC) in the brains of the participants when they viewed the photographs of the healthy faces. This part of the brain is associated with the assessment of risk and fear as well as decision-making. It has also been shown that the vmPFC plays a role in regulating the amygdala, the cluster of neurons deep in the cerebrum that, among other functions, triggers the fight or flight response. The increased vmPFC activity when looking at the pictures of healthy faces, then, is an indication that the absence of infection has been detected and communicated to the part of the brain responsible for determining the level of safety. Our elemental impulse to escape – our default mode, as it were – has been overridden. We're safe, it is saying. This person is healthy. No need to flee. This all happens in an instant, of course, without any awareness of the stimulus or its interpretation. On the level of conscious thought, we merely see the face of a sick person as less 'likeable', and the only explanation the brain will offer for this decision is 'instinct'. This is all a remnant, though, of the original evolutionary steps that helped early humans be conscious of their own state of health and take steps to maintain it so as to have the best possible chance of survival.

Beyond the adaptations that formed this detection-and-response aspect of the behavioural immune system developed yet another line of defence against potential infection. These were precautionary behaviours – steps that could be taken to minimise the risk of harm from disease before its presence was even confirmed, even on a subconscious level. A whole suite of psychological systems emerged to assess and manage the probability of potential threats according to the circumstances. These consisted of a coordinated set of mechanisms that both took in new feedback about likely threats and drew on memory to make associations with past events. In this way, early warning signs could be acted on and probabilities accounted for. If the presence of what experts have called a 'threat-signalling cue' was noted, a cascade of subsequent behaviours would follow. Thus, if an individual with a skin rash arrived, and the observer had previous experience of such rashes developing into a serious or fatal illness, they would likely shun or even actively reject any close contact with the rash-bearer without waiting for conformation that the same illness was present this time. Over time, shortcuts develop: any kind of skin problem will trigger the impulse to avoid contact, as might the arrival of a stranger who could be bringing new pathogens into the community. These threat management systems, whether focused on disease, violence or other potential dangers, are all biased against taking risk of any kind. There's a sense of 'better safe than sorry' running through all the research on this topic. The brain is aware that the system can produce errors, such as instinctively avoiding food that may well be completely fine to eat, but the perception of the costs involved in potentially eating something contaminated far outweigh the short-term loss of taking the precaution.

There is a contradiction here, of course, one that is fundamental to the nature of hypochondria. The unimpeded function of these systems has been a vital part of human development and survival, but an overactive awareness and avoidance of threats can become a debilitating condition in its own right. If hypochondria is characterised by a fear of illness, then it follows that being highly sensitive to the threat of illness is a key part of the condition. Research bears this out: in a 2016 study, a similar experiment was performed with photographs of sick and healthy faces, and, compared with the control, participants with severe health anxiety were found to perceive healthy people as being significantly less healthy and attractive. All of those traits that have provided humans with evolutionary advantages – hesitation around the unfamiliar, wariness of disease, protective behaviours that reduce contagion and general risk aversion – are experienced at a much higher level by those with health anxiety. These sufferers have what the study's authors called 'hyperactive disease avoidant mechanisms'. In other words, for some of us, an excessive amount of these evolutionary advantages morphs into a baseless, involuntary and open-ended anxiety about health.

But to exist in this continual state of alertness, braced for every possible disaster regardless of how likely it is, can also undermine the very state of health it is intended to preserve. 'Hypervigilance' is the state of mind that is today often associated with anxiety about health – an enhanced awareness of both the body and the environment through which it moves. In this mode of being, any symptom or change in the body is perceived as being more dangerous than it likely is in reality, leading to the 'tendency grossly to overestimate the probability of becoming ill and the seriousness of the dreaded illness', as the psychologist Stanley Rachman put it. The precise direction that the hypervigilance takes depends on circumstances – someone living with the constant fear of a stroke will avoid different things from someone terrified that they are about to come down with food poisoning. Regardless of the form it takes, this constant involuntary monitoring of threats and symptoms can feel primal and instinctive, an ancient survival mechanism in our nature that has not quite adapted to the realities of the modern world.

Hypochondria may be a glitch in the human system, but it also offers a way to look sideways at the very concept of health. When we do so, it becomes clear that our health exists as a spectrum, not a binary: beyond 'kill or cure', there are so many other states of being. To understand how the ever-shifting boundaries of hypochondria were drawn, then, we need to go back to the start of medicine itself.

The oldest surviving medical records are from Ancient Egypt, among them the document known as the Kahun Gynaecological Papyrus. This dates from around 1800 BCE and was found in 1889 near the modern Egyptian city of Al Lahun, about sixty miles south of Cairo. It was obviously well used; aside from the wear and tear of passing centuries, the papyrus has been patched with a fragment of an administrative document from around the same time, suggesting that somebody repaired it to increase its longevity. It comprises thirty-four paragraphs about women's health, each a kind of medical triptych. They read like this:

> Examination of a woman aching in her molars, her front, and her ears so much that she hears no word
> You should say of it 'it is terrors of the womb'
> You should treat it with the same prescription used for removing detritus of the womb

In three blunt phrases, the author of the treatise addresses the imagined physician reader, instructing them how to approach their patient and what to say. Almost everything in this document can be traced back to the womb: all complaints are caused by 'discharges', 'terrors', 'wanderings', 'clenches' or 'pains' of that organ. In one standout passage, the papyrus states that a woman suffering from 'aching in her teeth and molars to the point that she cannot (open) her mouth' should be told that she is suffering from 'toothache of the womb' and needs to have 'the urine of an ass' poured over her body as a cure.

In both this document and the Edwin Smith Papyrus, which dates from around 1600 BCE although is believed to be a scribe's copy of a text written around a thousand years earlier, we get only the physician's perspective, not that of the patient. We have no way of telling whether any of the women described felt satisfied with the womb-based explanation of their discomfort, although I like to imagine that the person receiving the 'toothache' diagnosis would seek a second opinion if she could. There are no other surviving documents that deal with this, so there is no more contemporary information on women's health and treatment with which to cross-reference, but it is still striking that the wide variety of complaints in the Kahun Papyrus – including problems with eyes, teeth, ears and legs – are, without exception, diagnosed as somehow caused by the womb. Again, we can't be sure, but it seems reasonable from what else we know about Egyptian society at this time to infer that the physicians treating these women were men; men who had never experienced the complaints their patients described and found the same explanation viable for such a variety of physical problems. Even at the very beginning, healthcare was rife with inequities, with more care taken of some people than others.

The Edwin Smith Papyrus, by contrast, is a surgical treatise, detailing how to diagnose visible and mechanical failures of the body like fractures, breaks and wounds. Reading it provides some heady jolts of recognition; its advice is fundamentally similar to the way such issues might be treated today – it details that physicians should use their hands to feel where bones are misaligned and then apply splints and bandages to promote healing. When the problems with the body were mechanical and largely visible, the healers of over 3,000 years ago came to similar conclusions to those of today. Together, these documents provide a glimpse of an emerging method, a system for understanding health via the relationship between symptoms and treatment. A patient presents with a problem, and the physician uses the tools at hand (mostly their actual hands) to explore its extent and prescribe a treatment. The latter might involve donkey urine, crocodile dung, honey or goose fat, but it is recognisably part of the same process we follow today.

However, not all of the medical literature from this time fits so conveniently into this template, and that is where we get our first inklings of Ancient Egyptian hypochondria – even though we are still many centuries away from being able to call it that. The Ebers Papyrus is also dated to the second millennium BCE, the ink thought to have been applied to the scroll in around 1550 BCE, although its twenty metres of script may also be a copy of a much earlier text. It gives a wonderfully broad view of Egyptian medicine and provides evidence that many of the conditions that humans still suffer from and puzzle over – depression, dementia, asthma – were already the subject of much concern over 3,000 years ago. Upon first reading, it appears to be a document at war with itself, though. On the one hand, it reflects the burgeoning empiricism also on display in the Edwin Smith and Kahun Papyri; an established recognition of the chain of cause and effect between symptoms, disease and treatment. But on the other hand, it is a highly superstitious document, containing around 700 remedies and incantations that can be deployed against a whole panoply of sicknesses. Belief alone in the power of these remedies justifies their use. As one Egyptologist in the 1930s put it, this text is 'medical and magical throughout'.

To understand why a culture that was comfortable with something approaching a scientific method would also prioritise spells and incantations as a part of maintaining health, it is necessary to consider how disorders might have been experienced at this time when there was no way whatsoever to see within the body, either literally or figuratively, to understand what might be going wrong. Unlike broken bones and postpartum injuries, much of the Ebers Papyrus deals with those 'subtle mysterious disturbances' to health that the physician cannot see with the eyes or feel with the hand, and with conditions that might be producing visible effects, like weight loss, skin discoloration or sweating, but for which no cause can be discerned. For the Egyptians of this time, there was little or no difference between these two types of impairment, observable and invisible. Just like a broken bone, an indeterminate illness is a risk to life, and the primary aim of the physician is to examine the symptoms, make a diagnosis and devise a course of treatment. If the cause of an unseen internal illness can be attributed to some unseen force – such as an evil spirit – then it follows that the physician must treat it by enlisting the help of a goddess such as Aset, or Isis, to rid the afflicted body of the malevolent presence. Only once it has been banished can remedies made from plants and animal products be used to repair the damage left behind. In some cases gods are listed as the original authors of the remedies included in the papyrus;

in others a specific prayer is given that must be said over the raw ingredients of a treatment to give it the desired curative power when they are mixed together. One memorable entry on treating 'tremors of the fingers' prescribes a concoction that includes 'excrement of the gods' as well as caraway, wax, honey and figs; quite how the physician is supposed to obtain this holy dung is not explained.

The implications of this for what we now consider to be hypochondria are profound. As far as we know, this is the earliest indication of a systematic understanding of health and medicine, and within it the apparently contradictory powers of science and magic are completely merged. Many centuries later, the role of belief or 'magical thinking' in the experience of health would become a major focus of stigma and then research. Today, three questions underpin our understanding of hypochondria. Is the patient *really* ill, or do they just believe themselves to be sick? Is the problem truly in and of their body, or have they concocted it with their mind? And does the treatment work because it intrinsically alters something on a cellular level, or does it work because the patient believes in its power? The root of all these knotty problems can be found in the Ancient Egyptian medical texts of the second century BCE. The exact nature of the 'magic' or belief involved will change – we now put our trust in higher beings in the form of wellness influencers, nutritional gurus and superfood salespeople rather than fertility goddesses – but the notion that belief and a power beyond human knowledge influence our health and bodies remains with us.

After her husband John Gregory Dunne died from a sudden heart attack in 2003, the writer Joan Didion embarked on what she described as 'a year of magical thinking'. She could pinpoint its beginning precisely: this new epoch commenced on the first evening after his death. She spent that night alone in their New York apartment, despite attempts from friends and loved ones to join her in her nocturnal grief. The solitude was purposeful. The magic wouldn't work otherwise, she felt instinctively. 'I had to be alone so that he could come back,' she wrote a few months later. While she was by herself, she could keep all of the conventional activities that accompany a recent death at bay: the weeping, the relaying of the news, the funeral planning. She brought the bag of John's possessions home with her from the hospital where he had been pronounced dead on arrival and carefully put them away, even placing his mobile phone – which he would never need again – on his desk to charge. As long as she maintained a sense of continuity with how everything had been while John was alive, this horrible change still felt reversible.

In the memoir she wrote about the year that followed John's death, Didion recalled the details of many such rituals she performed as part of the magic that would keep her husband alive. She refused to read his obituaries. She prevaricated over donating his organs, because he would, of course, need them when he returned. Likewise, she could not bring herself to give away his shoes, in case he required them again. Even as she was arranging for his cremation and for his name to be added to a marble memorial plaque, she was holding these mundane aspects of John's life in limbo for him to reclaim. With hindsight, she can see the utter contradiction inherent in this – someone whose ashes have been interred will never need shoes again – but at the time, in the midst of the raw shock of early grief, it all made perfect sense to her.

'Magical thinking' is a general term that covers several different kinds of behaviour around cause and effect, but it is one way in which we can see the continuity of thought and habit around illness from the very earliest times to today. Anthropologists use this phrase to describe any ritual or religious practice that involves an action and an expected compensation, such as a sacrifice to a god that leads to a divine favour, or the incantations listed in the Ebers Papyrus that praise a god in return for imbuing an ingredient with the power to cure an illness. In psychology, it has a broader meaning related to a person's belief that their thoughts or actions can influence events that in reality have no link, such as Didion's insistence that if she did not read any of her husband's obituaries, he could still come back to life. In psychiatry, aspects of magical thinking are identified as symptoms of conditions like obsessive compulsive disorder and some personality disorders; the belief that repeatedly turning a light switch on and off a certain number of times will guarantee safety, for instance, is a classic example of this. Superstition can be a kind of magical thinking too, as seen in habits like avoiding walking under ladders or staying in a hotel room numbered thirteen in case this bad choice is repaid with some future harm. This is the type of thought pattern that I sometimes fell prey to while I was undergoing cancer treatment.

Like Didion, I fully understood the absurdity of what I was doing, and yet I would still make sure I avoided all the cracks in the pavement as I was walking to a crucial meeting with my doctor, believing that if I stepped on one he would have bad news for me. The cadence of the treatments I received pushed me in this direction, with long periods of chemotherapy in which no new information was forthcoming, and then one-off scans to check its effectiveness that suddenly provided huge amounts of new data about my health and chances of recovery. It was around these events that the magical thinking was most pronounced. In between lying in the machine and visiting the consultant to hear the results, I would look for signs in the clouds and the number of ladybirds on my windowsill that things would go my way, even though I also knew completely that they had absolutely no bearing on the news I would receive. At one crucial point in my illness, this cycle of thinking became so pervasive in the run-up to a results meeting that I took unnecessary cold medicine at night, just to stop me from counting and interpreting the shadows on the ceiling instead of sleeping.

As with many experiences during my time having cancer, this now feels like a rehearsal for the hypochondria that followed. When I am in the grip of an anxious episode, such as an imaginary lump or a period of inexplicable fatigue, I will look out to the rest of the world for indications that I can safely abandon my fears. During a long train journey once, I counted the telegraph poles I saw between each station and decided that if there was an even number, I was most likely going to be fine. Being able to hold these contradictory ideas in my head simultaneously – that random numbers have an influence over my body and the knowledge that they absolutely do not – feels very in sync with hypochondria. It is a form of doubt that is constantly reaching out for reassurance, no matter how absurd or illogical.

The first literary account of hypochondria comes not from Egypt but from the Babylonian Empire, which in the second millennium BCE occupied what is now modern-day Iraq. *Ludlul bēl nēmeqi*, or 'The Poem of the Righteous Sufferer', takes the form of a lengthy monologue from a nobleman who has endured a sequence of great calamities. He has been forsaken by both the gods and his fellow men, then struck down by a painful cocktail of mysterious illnesses: 'Debilitating Disease is let loose upon me,' he laments. His list of symptoms is prodigious: he has a headache, an 'evil cough', cramp, impotence, an aching neck and chest, convulsions, a fever, concussion and paralysis, and, in a touch that hints at a vital component of hypochondria for millennia afterwards, he proclaims that 'they upset my bowels'. This poem is thought to have been authored by the Babylonian courtier Šubši-mešrê-Šakkan, which would date it to the late second millennium BCE, although it is likely fiction rather than autobiography. As in the Ebers Papyrus, created in Ancient Egypt around the same time, the Sufferer blames his illnesses on a set of evil spirits that have come from all directions – the wind, the horizon, the mountains, the underworld – to plague him. It feels significant, too, that this first hypochondriac on the page gets to narrate their own story; unlike those nameless Egyptian women and their womb-based ailments, we are hearing of his travails first-hand.

He seeks treatment for his many ailments, only to find that his problems mystify the experts:

> My complaints have exposed the incantation priest,
> And my omens have confounded the diviner.
> The exorcist has not diagnosed the nature of my
>   complaint,
> Nor has the diviner put a time limit on my illness.

Like many a sufferer since, he is cut adrift from the certainties that the medicine of the time purports to offer. He is alone, held in limbo. He is in a state of pain that nobody else can discern, isolated by his anxieties.

Eventually, he is given relief. The Ancient Mesopotamian god Marduk dispatches an exorcist who is able to cure the

Sufferer, at which point he becomes something like a poster boy for the god's power: his fellow citizens, who had previously shunned him during his period of undetectable illness, burst forth with praise for Marduk's healing ways, and the poem ends as the Sufferer is blessed and feasted at the temple complex in Babylon. It becomes a morality tale, 'The Babylonian Pilgrim's Progress' as one writer put it, demonstrating what faith can do to alleviate suffering while also highlighting the uncomfortable truth that the divine figure allowed such suffering to occur in the first place. Reading it thousands of years later, another, somewhat unsettling, message filters through. The Sufferer seems to be telling us that when medicine cannot help you, only your belief in the divine will save you. Magic and medicine are utterly intertwined. The allegorical resonance of the poem makes it unlikely that it is drawn entirely from real life, although its survival over the centuries after it was composed suggests that details from its first-person description of a hypochondriac's redemption resonated with its Babylonian readers. It remained popular throughout the first millennium BCE, being reproduced and distributed on many different tablets.

Another text from this region, thought to date from the eighth century BCE and only discovered in 2008, gives us something just as rare: a non-fiction first-person account of hypochondria. The author is one Adad-bēl-ardi, ruler of a small area on the banks of the Upper Euphrates in Syria, who tells the tale of his lifelong maladies. From early childhood he has suffered with sores all over his body, along with headaches, blurred vision and aches in his hands. Offerings to the gods have not alleviated his suffering, nor have visits to the doctor or the exorcist. No unifying cause can be found for his disparate problems, and indeed the fact that in this era he survived well into adulthood to write about his symptoms strongly hints at his problems being at least partially mental rather than physical. Unlike the earlier poem, this document does not use stock phrases from well-known medicinal incantations to describe symptoms; the language is personal and specific, not professional or religious. 'This text is a description, in layman's words, of chronic illness which has afflicted the patient since childhood,' as one expert puts it. It is the case history of a hypochondriac deeply immersed in the mysteries of his body – obsessed by them, even – and perpetually dissatisfied by the insufficient explanations of his doctors. Whether Adad-bēl-ardi's condition would have been curable by a later doctor is irrelevant; his experience was that of hypochondria because the expertise of the time had nothing more concrete to offer him than the suggestion that it might all be in his head. As with 'The Poem of the Righteous Sufferer', the crucial tension is between the patient's experiences of their condition and the lack of an explanation from the medical authorities.

It feels necessary to believe that medicine only moves in one direction, towards making us feel better, not worse. That the light of reason gradually burns ever brighter, making the murky shadows of misunderstanding and superstition retreat further into the corners. But this is not how progress, or indeed humanity, works. Some of the ideas implemented thousands of years ago by Hippocrates and his disciples are still consistent with today's science, such as using traction to realign broken bones before allowing them to heal in position, and promoting regular physical exercise as part of a regimen aimed at maintaining a healthy body and mind. Others seem bizarre or even harmful to us now, like the therapeutic bleeding to 'cure' vertigo and prescribing regular sex to childless women to prevent their wombs being 'displaced'. In every age, there have been beliefs and treatments that are subsequently proved to be well-founded in science, and those that are not. Our best efforts and intentions do not turn uncertainty into certainty. The passage of time does not automatically turn imperfection into perfection.

I first learned this, grimly, during the meeting in which I was told I had cancer. In a coincidence so cloyingly symmetrical that it made my hackles rise in suspicion, after outlining his proposed treatment plan, my oncologist explained that he'd had the very same disease when he was a teenager. He had survived, and my experience was going to be so much better than his had been, he assured me. The generalised radiation and powerfully toxic chemotherapy he had endured were long gone, consigned to medical history, and replaced by much more targeted and effective care. He showed me the scar along his jawline as a kind of negative reassurance: you won't end up looking as bad as this, he suggested. He was right; my scars are the same size, but they are much less easy to see. Just last year, though, I received a letter from my local healthcare provider telling me that I was now at an elevated risk of breast cancer and must begin annual monitoring immediately. Scrabbling through the paperwork for an explanation for this out-of-the-blue declaration of danger, I discovered that new research had revealed that the radiotherapy I had received to eradicate tumours from my chest could actually make contracting this other form of cancer more likely. It felt like the validation of all my supposedly unfounded anxieties. Now I had a new worry: my cure might end up being the thing that kills me. But it was the best that could be done at the time to keep me alive.

Every act of ministering to our bodies is mired in this paradox. Everything is the best available option, a work in progress reflecting a partial but growing understanding of all the ways in which flesh and bone and brain can malfunction. But the illusion of certainty is vital to the smooth operation of modern medicine. In order to keep doing their jobs, doctors need to believe that what they are prescribing will do more good than harm. Patients similarly can't think too hard about this; would I have climbed into the radiation machine so calmly and stood so completely still while invisible particles were fired at my torso if I had known about the misery that doing so might lead to in the future? I would like to believe that I would, but perhaps that is to overestimate my courage. I allowed myself to be reassured by my doctor. He gave me a measure of peace along with the toxic chemicals that shrunk my tumours and made all my hair fall out. At no point during the process did he make me feel like I was just another insignificant data point in a vast and ongoing science experiment, even though that is exactly what I was. What I still am.

Being a hypochondriac can sometimes feel like I alone can see the wires holding it all up. As if the rest of the world operates cheerfully on the basis that medicine is infallible and can offer absolute certainty, and only I realise that it is all an approximation based on the best evidence that we have right now. As though everyone else is happily inhabiting the simulation and only I am aware of the code streaming through the air that shapes reality. This is just one of many rationalisations I use to justify my fears, of course. The fact that the latest medicine is merely the most recent iteration of ongoing research does not detract from its essential, critical role in society. In every aspect of life, we do the best that we can with what we have at any given moment. These words I am writing now are all that I have this morning; who knows if you will read them in the eventual book. Perhaps I will be able to do better tomorrow. Improvement, even by the smallest possible increments, is the opposite of failure. But when fear inclines us to doubt, it feels like only certainty can quiet the panic. And hard as it is to confront this idea, there is no such thing as certainty when it comes to our health, nor will there ever be.

2

All Disease Begins in the Gut

Until the fifth century BCE, the word 'hypochondria' did not exist, and even then it would be over a thousand years before the condition as we know it now would be called by that name. That said, there are traces of symptoms and behaviours we now associate with hypochondria to be found in the ancient world. Cicero, in the book he penned while in mourning for his beloved daughter, writes of those who are prone to 'a continual anxiety' about the potential for future illness: 'We say that some people are rheumatic, others dropsical, not because they are so at present, but because they are often so: some are inclined to fear, others to some other perturbation.' He used the Latin word *aegritudo* to refer to this anxiety, a term for illness used in medical textbooks – giving an official flavour to his observations. Philosophy of the classical period was greatly preoccupied with the propensity for dread of future harms – of all kinds, from illnesses to travel problems – to damage one's quality of life in the present. The Greek Cyrenaic school of the fourth century BCE developed a spiritual exercise to combat it that came to be known as *futurorum malorum præmeditatio,* during which you anticipate and visualise the worst possible future adversity so as to release yourself from the anxiety of dreading it. 'Ruminating beforehand upon future evils which you see at a distance makes their approach more tolerable,' Cicero declared approvingly. This technique was picked up and popularised by the Stoic philosophers of the first and second centuries CE and even now forms part of modern cognitive behavioural treatment for health anxiety, under the name 'negative visualisation'.

The first instance of the word 'hypochondria' itself crops up in Greece, in a collection of medical texts known as the Hippocratic Corpus. But, rather than being a term connected with the condition, 'hypochondria' is the label for a particular location within the body. The Corpus is associated with the work of, but not necessarily written by, the so-called father of medicine, the physician Hippocrates of Kos. In *Epidemics*, it is recorded that a woman who has recently given birth is suffering with pain in her right υποχόνδριος, or 'hypochondrion'. Once again, the connection with the female body is present from the beginning. The term crops up again in *Aphorisms*, another work from the Corpus, where it states that:

> Jaundice supervening, in fever, on the seventh, ninth, eleventh and fourteenth day is favourable: but if the right hypochondrium be indurated, it is not so.

Later in the same text we are told that 'milk is injurious to those who are afflicted with headache, fever, and distention of the hypochondrium' and that 'pains in the hypochondrium, unattended with inflammation, are relieved by fever'.

This is anatomical language, the words that allow us to give figurative shape to guts and gore. For Hippocrates, 'hypochondria' is a collective noun for the contents of the 'hyperchondrion' or 'hyperchondrium'. The geographical clue as to where this is situated in the body is in the components of the word itself: *hupo* meaning 'under' and *khondros* denoting the cartilage of the sternum in the original Greek. It describes the place where hard ribs give way to soft abdomen, where the liver, spleen and gall bladder nestle within our flesh. The interplay of ideas about these different organs and their location in the hyperchondrium would influence the direction of medicine for centuries to come.

Hypochondria at the time of Hippocrates, then, was merely a way for one physician to tell another where something was occurring in a patient's body. And this meaning of the word lingered for over 2,000 years, notwithstanding the way it overlapped and fused with later developments and definitions. When one Samuel Field of Deerfield, Massachusetts, was shot during an altercation with a Native American tribe in 1725, a chronicler described his injury thus: 'The ball passing through the right Hypochondria, cutting off three plaits of the mysenteria; a gut hung out of the wound in length almost two inches.' Surprisingly, given the state of surgery and aftercare at the time, Field did not die of this gruesome tear in his hypochondria; according to the same account he was fully healed after five weeks and lived another forty years, passing away at the age of eighty-three. Had Hippocrates himself been writing up the case history, he would have used the same language to denote where the wound was located. How could eighteenth-century colonists in North America still be using the same anatomical terms as the Ancient Greeks? While Hippocrates was groundbreaking in many of his observations, much of his language has long since been translated and assimilated into English medical vocabulary in diluted or modified forms. We no longer say, as he did, πνεύμονος, or 'pneúmōnos', to mean 'lungs', for instance. Yet hypochondria has come down to us unchanged, unscathed by the intervening millennia.

The appearance of the word 'hypochondria' in the Hippocratic Corpus was part of something much bigger that was happening to the practice of medicine as a result of a seismic shift in how health was understood. Prior to the widespread adoption of the Hippocratic method, sufferers would visit a shrine to Asclepius and make an offering, like an animal sacrifice or a petition carved onto a votive tablet. The priests would prescribe a course of treatments, such as bloodletting or a particular diet, with which the pilgrim could make themselves fit for divine intervention. They then had to sleep in the vicinity of the shrine – some of the larger complexes had extensive dormitories full of semi-permanent residents for this reason – and hope that the god they sought would appear to them in a dream with a cure. Although some aspects of this survived into the next phase of medicine and beyond (the specific techniques practised by the priests, for instance, and the 'health spa' ambience of the shrines), the whole system was underpinned by ritual and deference to divine visitation.

With the advent of the Hippocratic movement, superstition and belief were peeled away. 'There is not, in the entire Corpus, the slightest hint that disease is traceable to causes beyond the powers of the physician to understand,' as one medical historian puts it. Gone are the appeals to Isis or, more locally, the Greek god Asclepius, son of Apollo and father of among others Hygieia, goddess of health. Now medicine was a discipline that focused on natural and observable causes of disease only, and which saw nature itself as the source of all knowledge about health.

The central hypothesis of this school of medicine stated

that the body's natural state is one of stability, with all forces and constituent parts in balance. If an imbalance develops, this causes sickness. A physician can promote health in his patients by advocating a lifestyle and diet that maintain bodily balance, and also by prescribing treatments to correct deficits or excesses should they arise. Everything should be done to assist nature in curing itself. Hippocratic medicine also puts the patient at the centre of everything, rather than making the person actually suffering the sickness subordinate to the invisible forces of the universe, as in the Egyptian and Babylonian traditions.

The Hippocratic tradition advocated keeping the patient under close observation so as to be able to detect and correct the causes of disease. Scrutinising and tasting urine samples; listening to the sounds of the lungs; examining emissions like phlegm, mucus and diarrhoea; and observing fluctuations in the patient's skin colour and temperature were all central to the diagnostic process. Doctors following this protocol examined their patients physically, but of course, they could only inspect the parts they could see or feel, as the dissection of human bodies was taboo. The act of cutting through the skin of a patient was considered particularly sacrilegious as unbroken skin symbolised physical and moral integrity, for both the individual and the community at large.

One later follower of Hippocrates, Diocles of Carystus, is thought to have carried out a number of dissections during the fourth century BCE, and of course the examination of warriors wounded in armed conflict allowed a glimpse of what lay beneath the skin without the physician having to cut through it. But largely this was an era in which the basic understanding of the human interior had to be augmented by Egyptian texts – drawing on the mummification process – and animal dissection. Aristotle, writing in around 350 BCE, was especially influential in speculating about the nature of human anatomy based on the observation of the organs of animals, whereas Hippocrates' approach to medicine was very much based on empirical knowledge of the surface of the body.

'To him medicine owes the art of clinical inspection and observation,' the medical historian Fielding Hudson Garrison wrote of Hippocrates in 1913. 'It is the method of Hippocrates, the use of the mind and senses as diagnostic instruments ... that makes him the greatest of all physicians.' Forty-two of his case histories survive, of which several, experts have said, could easily be reprinted today in a modern textbook without students noticing any major anomaly. His accounts of progressive illness and its symptoms are precise, honest and entirely lacking in self-aggrandisement. Death hovers very near in these texts: in twenty-five of these case histories the patient does not survive, which is hardly a great advertisement for a physician with an eye on attracting more paying clients. Hippocrates recorded their illnesses anyway, perhaps as a kind of testimonial, or perhaps hoping that others might one day succeed where he had failed.

In addition to establishing the fundamental structure for a medical history, Hippocrates' case notes also make for surprisingly moving reading. He notes that patients gripped by serious fever often tug and tear at their bedclothes when the 'crisis' of their illness approaches – a suddenly recognisable and human trait amid all of the impersonal enumeration of bodily fluids. One account, in particular, gave me a jolt of recognition:

In Thasus, a woman, of a melancholic turn of mind, from some accidental cause of sorrow, while still going about, became affected with loss of sleep, aversion to food, and had thirst and nausea.

I will never know the name of this woman who lived on this Greek island in the Aegean Sea 2,400 years before I was born, but I take some comfort from the knowledge that she, like me, was of a melancholic turn of mind that vented its fury upon her body. There is also something touching about the fact that her symptoms were so closely observed, that her suffering – whatever its cause – was seen, perhaps for the first time, by someone who knew how to properly look. This feels like a moment of profound vulnerability and a momentous step forward in how human beings thought about illness.

I stopped trying to destroy the photograph years ago. It was taken at a school dance when I was seventeen. I am wearing a long off-the-shoulder dress, although the picture was tightly framed and shows me from the neck upwards only. My friend Dave's grinning face occupies the left side of the image. We are dancing, throwing ourselves around as we slowly shed the self-consciousness of our earlier teenage years. Someone, I don't know who, clicked their camera right in our faces while we were in motion, stamping that moment onto paper. I first saw this picture when an envelope of developed shots from the party was passed round at school the following week. Later, it was scanned and sent to me digitally. Even though I've deleted it dozens of times, from every folder and email and hard drive where it has ever appeared, the shadow still exists. A ghostly image that only I can see. I look happy. My hair, which was then, pre-chemotherapy, thick and lank and straight, had been painstakingly twirled into bouncy ringlets. The broad red straps of the sparkly dress my cousin made for the occasion are just visible. I'm smiling, breathless and shiny from the exertion of dancing. I haven't yet found the tennis-ball-sized lump just above my left collarbone. And yet, in the photograph, it's already big enough to cast its own shadow on my neck.

How could I not have seen it then? How long had it been there?

The hypochondriac searches always for the first twinge, the first sensation, the first symptom, but that moment of awareness is not necessarily the true beginning of a disease. A tumour might have a billion cells before it intrudes upon our notice. An intruder, like a virus, bacterium or parasite, can lie dormant or even operate for years without making its host conscious of its presence. The body is hard to reckon with: it is intimately present and completely absent at the same time. I exist inside it and yet I cannot know what is happening within. As such, the hardest kind of disease for me to comprehend is one that is created of the same stuff as me. 'The creation of a tumour is an extraordinarily slow process, often extending over decades,' explains the cancer geneticist Robert A. Weinberg. 'The cells forming a tumour are all lineal descendants of a single progenitor, a distant ancestor that lived many years before the tumour mass became apparent. This founder, this renegade cell, decided to go off on its own, to begin its own growth programme within one of the body's tissues.' The original cell that starts the process might have existed, in some sense of that word, as long as I have. Living with this knowledge requires me to accept that I have no control over what happens to me or inside me, that my billions of cells do not work to my command or even for my attention. No amount of hypervigilance to my body's activities or changes will alert me to the fact that something has gone wrong earlier. I cannot study harder, or do better, or improve at this. It is merely a fact of being alive. And this is a very uncomfortable realisation.

Popular culture, especially fiction, teaches us that there is a moment of genesis, a beginning to the narrative of an illness, even if we cannot feel it. A historical romance novel that I read over and over in my teens retold the tale of sixteenth-century courtier Robert Dudley and his wife Amy Robsart, who was found dead in suspicious circumstances with a broken neck at the bottom of the stairs, thus blighting her husband's political career because the claustrophobic world of the Elizabethan court could never quite accept that he hadn't pushed her. Throughout the book, the writer mentions that Amy suffered from a pain in her breast, which she thought was the physical manifestation of the heartbreak her husband caused her. To the modern reader, though, this was clearly a foreshadowing of the cancer that experts have suggested could have contributed to her death, the accompanying osteoporosis having made her bones weak and fragile. The author confirms this in a note at the end of the book, making it clear that the reader has witnessed the private development of Amy's illness, even while she was not aware of it. Medical thrillers like Robin Cook's *Terminal* go even further into this, using an omniscient narrator to pinpoint the exact moment that ordinary cells mutate, unbeknown to the person in whose head they reside. The television drama *House* often uses a similar device as part of the show's visual language, zooming impossibly into the microscopic level within the suddenly transparent body of a patient with a mysterious condition and showing computer-animated sequences of cells dividing or nerves fusing. This is entirely science fiction, as unlike the reality of even the most cutting-edge medical science as the comic strip I used to read as a child about 'the Numskulls', who were a collection of miniature technicians that lived inside a person's head and controlled the various functions of their body, usually to comically disastrous effect. We cannot see or feel or know the moment at which an illness or a disorder begins. And yet we remain obsessed with the idea that perhaps we can. The lure of narrative overrides the mere knowledge that science can offer.

If I had to isolate the precise moment that hypochondria reared up from somewhere inside and took hold of me, it would not be when the doctor said I had cancer, nor when my mother fainted in shock at his words and slid off her chair. It was afterwards, when he was examining me and asking questions so that he could create a treatment plan. He gestured at my neck, his eyes dropping briefly from my face to look at the area just above my left collarbone. 'Other than that one,' he said, gesturing to the place, 'have you noticed any other masses?' The part of my body that he was referring to went instantly numb as I took in his words. I had not even noticed this mass, but it was certainly there now. It had grown so slowly, cell by cell, so gradually distending the skin of my neck that I had not registered the changes it was causing. I had so successfully conceptualised myself as a brain in a jar that something so fleshy had passed me by. Later, friends at school mentioned casually that they had noticed the lump but hadn't said anything because they assumed I already knew about it, because how could I not? How could I not? I turned the question over and over in my mind in the days that followed. That is the gap into which all of my anxiety bloomed. It is one thing to coexist with a disease that has yet to produce any discernible symptoms, and quite another to live months into its palpable, physical effects without realising what is happening. This is the reason that the photograph of me at the school dance still lingers so persistently for me, because it is visual proof that I had been sick for so much longer than I realised. For months, I had been putting my constant tiredness and distraction down merely to the pressure of university entrance tests and interviews, assuming that it was all tension created by my mind. I never gave my body a second thought; it never occurred to me that there might be some deeper wrongness at the root of it all. Now, I can never rid myself of the idea that something might be there, lurking in plain sight, if only I can find the right way of looking for it.

This feels like a rational response to me. I have shared my body with a dangerous intruder without realising it before, so it constantly feels possible that this has happened again. I also know with hindsight that this cohabitation had mental, as well as physical, effects, so nothing I experience is off limits from this constant examination for potential danger. During those months that the tumours were expanding inside me without me knowing it, I withdrew from some of my closest friendships and stopped taking an interest in hobbies I had previously cared deeply about. Again, I and everyone around me attributed the new, world-weary filter on my previously eager and earnest personality as merely the changes that come with growing up. Now I wonder if this mental shift, too, was a consequence of the cancer. It felt like I was turning in on myself, shutting the rest of the world out even as it faded into grey around me. As if all of my energy was being consumed by something within.

If I allow myself, I can get lost in the endless loop of these thoughts. How long had the cancer cells been an invisible passenger on my journey through teenagehood? Perhaps they were present for my first kiss, the first time I drove a car, the first time a scene I wrote was performed in front of a real audience. Dwell on this too long and I begin to connect more and more memories to my illness. I remember the sunny September Sunday when I was eleven years old, when my family was spending the afternoon cutting the golden brown meadow grass at the bottom of the garden, and I said I felt too unwell to help so that I could lie in bed and read a book instead. Had it already begun then, this melding of my self with the sickness? Is it happening again, right now? There is no answer that will ever satisfy me; there will always be something I can't yet know, can't yet see, or haven't yet seen. And it's in that gap of uncertainty that the worries lie. Where there is room for doubt, the hypochondriac sets about filling it with supposition.

The seeds of doubt from which modern-day hypochondria grew were present even during the rationalist revolution in Greece in the fifth and fourth centuries BCE. Hippocrates is credited with laying the scientific foundations of modern healthcare, but his methods and those of his contemporaries were not entirely free from superstition. Even though very few people had ever actually looked inside a human body, they did not consider it to be a blank, unknowable space. What went on within was subject to a complex theoretical system which governed everything about how physicians and patients alike behaved. As a person relentlessly schooled in the modern requirement for theories to be backed up by observation and proper sources, it is perplexing to me that it could be so. 'Citation needed,' my brain keeps protesting as I immerse myself in this era of medical theory. Why didn't they want to *know* what was really going on inside?

The answer, of course, is that they did know. Or at least they thought they did, which is functionally the same thing. Just as I think I have a decent working knowledge of how my organs are laid out, based on the research I have done and all the various scans of my insides that I have seen, the Hippocratic physicians felt similarly confident that they had the right of it. This has been an unexpected lesson I've learned while writing this story: no knowledge of the body is final. We are an ever-updating mass of versions and theories, and any sense of certainty is an illusion. It makes me think of the long-exposure photography of the artist Alexey Titarenko, who in the early 1990s walked around his home city of St Petersburg on long winter nights and captured the movement that he observed with a long exposure time and a slow shutter speed. His 'people-shadows' have blurred outlines created by the infinitesimally different versions superimposed upon each other. In one particularly memorable shot, a mother and child are walking towards the lens, the shape of their dark coats static while their faces are exploding from the collars in an incomprehensible mass of contradiction. This is how I have come to visualise the human body – an entity built out of elusive, ever-altering layers of understanding. At any given time, we are looking at both what we know for sure now and everything we have known before, while future certainties not yet understood hover around the edges.

The body in the time of Hippocrates was a hectic place. It was a meeting point for all of the opposing forces in the universe, which needed to stay in balance for a good state of health to be maintained. In the Hippocratic tradition, the body is constituted of four humours – a term derived in part from the Greek word ὑγρός, or *humon*, meaning fluid or wet. Phlegm, yellow bile, black bile and blood were thought to originate in the liver and the stomach. These elemental liquids were forged in the heat of the human digestive process and then moved around the body, where they were ultimately consumed by the flesh – a one-way, rather than circulatory, system. One of my favourite explanations of this system comes from a 1970s paper: 'From earliest times doctors theorised that life consists of juices. The body was only the container in which the juices flowed,' it declares. Life is juicy: a brief motto that somehow manages to bind together the wet, squishy vulnerability of human existence with an irrepressible optimism about what we might manage to do here before we expire.

Temperature and moisture were the foundational characteristics of these juices; their combination gave each humour its nature. Phlegm was cold and wet, yellow bile was hot and dry, black bile was cold and dry, and blood was hot and wet. Beyond this, each humour had a whole host of compatible associations, including a season, an element, a temperament, an astrological sign, a body type and a propensity for particular diseases. People were usually born with an inclination towards or away from a certain humour, depending on the unique balance of fluids within their body. Environment and habit could also have an impact on the balance of humours. Thus, someone with an excess of phlegm is connected to the element of water, the season of winter and 'water signs' like Pisces and Aquarius, while an excess of yellow bile denotes fire, summer and 'dry' signs like Virgo and Leo. Together, the humours form what was known as a *mixis*, which in turn affected the *complexion*, or state of health. When all four were in balance, the body was healthy. Disease occurred when there was a deficit or excess of one or more humours, and any treatment applied would act to bring everything back into harmony.

Hippocrates did not entirely invent this system for interpreting the universe and our place within it – aspects of it can be found in writing by Homer, Aristotle and Pythagoras as well as in Egyptian and Babylonian texts – but it is in a work from the Hippocratic Corpus, *On the Nature of Man*, that the theory is most clearly described and codified. Zany as it seems now, especially when connected with a figure generally lauded for his influence on the scientific method, humoral theory does at least offer an attractively holistic way to understand life and health. Even personality differences could be explained by the state of someone's humours: someone with an excess of hot and dry yellow bile, for instance, would be quick-tempered and argumentative, while too much cold black bile would imply sluggishness, introspection and a tendency to depression. It is easy to see the appeal of this. The complex web of associations and imbalances has an answer for everything, and it is all rooted in something everybody is familiar with – the body. As one historian puts it, it provides 'a continuum between passions and cognition, physiology and psychology, individual and environment'. It is a bastion against the terror of the unknown. It explains everything.

The incredibly tenacious influence of this system for thinking about health can even be discerned today in the language that we use to describe people of different temperaments. If we say that someone is sanguine, we mean that they are even-tempered or even optimistic – traits that belong to the airy, spring-like humoral condition of excess blood, or sanguinity. A choleric individual is quick-tempered and irritable, as per the fiery temperament associated with yellow bile, or *choler*. Even the word 'humour' itself has retained its association with balance and a healthy outlook on life; on a good day I might be in good humour, and on a bad day lacking in it.

Perhaps the most difficult aspect of humoral theory to comprehend, but the most important for understanding how it is intertwined with the history of hypochondria, is the fact that the humours were figurative rather than observable. Although they were conceptualised as fluids and based upon visible substances, nobody expected to be able to cut into the body and fill a vial with pure black bile. The blood that demonstrably filled human veins was not the same as the humoral ideal of blood, or *haima*, nor was the mucus that ran out of the nose during a cold entirely composed of humoral phlegm, *phlegmos*. The humours did not need to be tangible to live in the imagination. They were metaphorical entities, the product of a meeting between body and mind to create something that was of both and of neither. These insubstantial bodily fluids explained everything in a perfect loop of logic. The body was inherently composed of and governed by the humours, therefore anything that went wrong with the body was caused by them – a confirmation of the theory.

Before the development of more empirical techniques for understanding the body, similar systemic notions of corporeal equilibrium emerged in plenty of cultures. The classical Ayurveda texts of the Indian subcontinent have a similar focus on holistic treatments and bodily balance, while the five elements of Chinese medicine – wood, water, earth, metal and fire – play a comparable role to humours, with the bodily organs, fluids and senses as well as the terrestrial seasons organised according to this scheme. Yin and yang must be in balance in the body for health to be maintained; a yin deficiency will result in overheating, dryness and muscular tension, while not enough yang will make the body cold and clammy. As in the Hippocratic tradition, imbalance is treated with a rebalancing regime of diet and exercise – 'warm' foods like turmeric, ginger and chestnuts might be prescribed to help a cold body return to equilibrium, for example.

Given the prominent role that the liver played in humoral theory as the origin of the humours, and the fact that this organ occupied the part of the body known at this time as the 'hypochondria', a close association existed between the two. Black bile, in particular, was inextricably linked to this term and this part of the body, being made in the liver but stored in the spleen – another hypochondriac organ. Cold and dry, this humour was associated with autumn, afternoon, sluggishness and depressive personalities. The Greek term for this humour, *melaina chole*, literally translates as 'black bile' and is also the root of the word 'melancholy'. A constitution that was inclined to exhibit an excess of black bile was more likely to develop melancholia, a condition that Hippocrates characterised as 'a fright or despondency [that] lasts for a long time' and included symptoms such as 'aversion to food, despondency, and insomnolency; irritability, restlessness'. This was both a mental and physical condition: a psychological state born of a physiological imbalance or disease in the hypochondria. And in a hint of what was to come, melancholy was already acknowledged as an unreliable and hard-to-pin-down consequence of humoral imbalance. As one expert puts it, 'an excess of black bile did not necessarily give rise to identifiable illnesses'. Some melancholics experienced only 'natural, nonpathogenic' symptoms, and even found the state conducive to inspiration. From the start, melancholy was a mystery closely intwined with hypochondria as we understand it today – and it was one that thinkers were about to spend the next 2,000 years trying to solve.

Although the four humours were to remain the default explanation for any bodily malfunction for more than a thousand years after the death of Hippocrates himself, the thinking around them wasn't entirely static. Subsequent physicians and medical theorists both in Greece and elsewhere were constantly revising and tweaking the theory, adding new associations for each humour and elaborating on the nature of the human body. One of these updates, proposed by Diocles of Carystus in around 350 BCE, was to prove especially consequential for hypochondria. For the first time, the hypochondria was no longer just an anatomical region or a place for storing black bile, but connected to a real ailment.

Diocles hypothesised that there was a connection between the organs of the hypochondrium, a particular kind of melancholy and blockages in the digestive system. 'Some call it melancholic, others flatulent,' he writes, before entering into what could easily be a description of what we might today colloquially call an 'upset stomach' or a 'bad tummy'. There will be 'a burning feeling near the hypochondrium', pains in the back or belly, a gurgling noise and, if unlucky, the vomiting of undigested food. The proximity and close connection between the hypochondrium and the stomach, as well as the former's pre-existing link to black bile and melancholy, unite in this one affliction. This was to prove an extremely long-lasting connection; it is still the case today that many hypochondriacs are focused on their digestion, whether in the form of a condition like irritable bowel syndrome, a morbid fear of unexplained vomiting, or some other intestinal complaint.

Around the time that Diocles made the connection between the digestive system and physical disorders in the hypochondrium section of the abdomen, Plato theorised that this area where the liver resided was the seat of an important part of the soul in the human body. In the *Timaeus*, he declared:

> That part of the soul which desires meats and drinks and the other things of which it has need by reason of the bodily nature, they placed between the boundary of the navel ... and there they bound it like a wild animal that was chained up with man.

This combination of the digestive and the emotional was fundamental to being human, Plato went on. In a healthy, morally virtuous person, the 'natural sweetness of the liver' and the bitter substance that it produced, black bile, balanced each other out. If all was well, this soul-liver would be 'happy and joyful', enabling restful sleep and even, in special cases, divinely inspired prophetic dreams. The spleen, another soul-infused organ that inhabited part of the hypochondrium region, existed to keep the liver bright and pure, 'like a napkin, always ready prepared and at hand to clean the mirror'.

The influence of Plato's theories, combined with the burgeoning Hippocratic tradition within medicine, was profound. The hypochondrium thus became the site of two seemingly unrelated processes within the body: digestive function and emotional disorder. This was underlined by the work of Galen of Pergamon, a second century CE Greek physician who practised medicine in Rome and was a personal physician to several emperors. He built on the digestive and emotional connections made by his forebears, but emphasised the crucial role that black bile played in causing anxiety in a patient. Even its hue was highly significant for him:

> For just as darkness outside causes fear in all people ... likewise the colour of black bile very similarly casts a shadow over the place where thinking is located, and produces fearing.

Galen goes on to itemise the signs that something more than just a bad reaction to food is present: symptoms in the stomach that are 'accompanied by melancholic affections', as well as 'despondency and fear'. When all of these are present, 'we call this disease hypochondriac and flatulent,' he says.

By the second century CE, then, the transition away from 'hypochondria' as a purely anatomical term is complete. It is now inextricably connected with a disease: one with physical symptoms, a suggested course of treatment – Galen recommends 'laxatives, emetics, breaking wind, and belching' – and a mental state that includes a propensity towards depression and anxiety.

Many of the changes that hypochondria would undergo in subsequent centuries are concerned with this combination of physical and mental, tangible and intangible. Today, we think of the separation between body and mind as that between the head and the rest of the person, but it all began much lower down, in the abdomen, where the digestive and hypochondriac organs inhabit the upper abdomen. That image from Plato of the soul as a wild animal chained in the liver, shackled both to our potential for virtue and the tools for good digestion, has haunted me ever since I first encountered it. This is the root of everything that hypochondria was to later become.

A strong cultural association remains between the digestive system and our emotional state, even for those who have no experience of hypochondria: we still talk of having a 'gut feeling' or 'going with my gut'. When we talk of the fluttery feeling of butterflies accompanying a moment of high anxiety or nerves, it is in the stomach region that we feel them flying. This sense of an instinctive understanding rooted in the abdominal area, separate from more 'rational' knowledge housed in the brain, is a survivor from this era of medical theory. It is also a key component of hypochondria. I can know logically that my every shiver is not the arrival of a fever, nor my every sneeze an indication that I have caught a deadly virus, but when the anxiety overrides this rational certainty it can feel like a different part of me is in charge, that my sensible brain is no longer in the driving seat. It is in the stomach region that I experience those ungovernable lurches of fear, as if that is still where the hypochondria rests within me, just as those Ancient Greek practitioners believed.

*

The body has what has been described as 'a limited vocabulary of subjective sensations'. I may think that I can feel things growing inside me that shouldn't be there, like roots creeping unseen through the soil, but there is no evidence to suggest that this is actually the case. A disproportionate amount of what we perceive on a visceral level as 'health' or the lack of it, I think, is to do with digestion. We are essentially tubes into which we put food to be processed every day; the limbs are just how we move the tubes around the world. Food's progress through us is responsible for many of the quotidian cues that tell us 'how we feel'. Digestive problems can produce all manner of sensations beyond the expected cramps and bloating. Food sensitivities can result in rashes, joint pain, fatigue and headaches, and trapped wind can be so painful that it has been known to send people to hospital emergency departments fearing that something inside them is about to rupture. And yet this complex inner process is something which we are culturally programmed to try to keep to ourselves. I remember once staying in a hotel that had assigned seating for breakfast, and I sat there morning after morning listening to the conversation of the family at the next table as they updated each other on their digestive sensations and bowel movements overnight. I found this practice fascinating and the conversations compelling in a way that is slightly uncomfortable to admit. They shared the contents of their insides casually and inquired after the minor ailments and curiosities of previous days with what sounded like genuine interest. It was how they expressed love for each other, I think. It made me think about the customary British formal greeting of 'how do you do?', to which the appropriate response is also 'how do you do?', not a description of how you are actually doing. I wonder what the world would be like if we were all absolutely honest in answering that question.

Digestion and stomach issues have come up a lot in my conversations with hypochondriacs over the years. They are often the focus of fears and symptoms; a severe aversion to vomiting is a common focus of health anxiety, as is food poisoning. One young woman I spoke to described how she had been mortally afraid of eating something that made her sick for years, to the extent that the idea of eating anything unfamiliar or trying new restaurants caused great anxiety. When in a new place, whether an unfamiliar country or just a different restaurant, food was always a source of worry. Perhaps this would be understandable had she had a serious gastric illness in the past and been anxious to avoid repeating the experience, but she had in fact never been unwell in this way before, and it was merely its possibility that had come to dominate her life. 'I almost wish I could just get food poisoning, you know,' she said, almost wistfully when we spoke, 'so that I would know for myself that it isn't that bad.' When I asked if she had a theory as to why this had become the focus of her hypochondria, she made an emotional, rather than physical or medical, connection to her past. 'I'm an only child of parents who really wanted children,' she explained. 'I was very loved and wanted when I was young, which is obviously great. But reflecting on it now, I think the fact that I was all they had made a difference. I wasn't aware of this connection at the time, but I think I became terrified that I would get sick from eating bad food and die, and I didn't want my parents to go through that, so I started being very careful about what I ate.'

The stomach is so connected to our emotional experiences. It clenches and flutters with excitement, feels hollow or twisted in nervousness, and lurches in shock. Queasiness or nausea is a common accompaniment to anticipation or uncertainty. I once went to bed for two days with what felt like a terrible stomach upset while I waited for someone who I knew was going to break up with me to get around to doing the deed. It wasn't until the dreaded conversation had finally happened and all my symptoms had abruptly ceased that I realised that I'd actually been immobilised by the clenching cramps of my own sadness. And there is now mounting evidence that the mix of microbes in the gut can influence the experience of mood disorders, anxiety and stress, as well as the response of the immune system. Research into this 'microbiota–gut–brain axis' is still in the early stages, and some critics question whether the results of studies that involved introducing so-called good bacteria into germ-free mice and then observing their lowered stress responses can be accurately read across to humans. Still, there are promising papers that hint of the impact a diverse gut microbiome can have on depression, anxiety and even perhaps some degenerative neurological diseases. Even while the science in this field advances, some of its findings are already trickling down to the consumer level, with probiotic supplements, recipe books offering 'good mood food' and dubious 'gut health' gurus already thriving. It all feels like a return to the very beginning of hypochondria: an emotional yet physical condition rooted in the abdomen that can be treated by the ingestion of the right food. About 2,500 years ago, Hippocrates declared, 'All disease begins in the gut', and modern science might well prove him right.

3

Sharp Belchings and Windy Melancholy

Is this normal? – the hypochondriac's perpetual refrain. Any slight alteration in the body or unexpected sensation is scrutinised through this lens. Should I have a bulge here, a tingle there, a crease between my eyes? So much of a hypochondriac's time and mental effort are taken up with this constant calculus as we try to determine whether fear is the correct response. Some seek medical advice for every little twinge, hoping that the expert will be able to put their feelings into a proper context. Others go in the opposite direction, avoiding all contact with doctors in case they deliver bad news, and instead look for their reassurance elsewhere, from loved ones or the internet. Whichever path we choose, the desired destination is the same. I want to be told that there is nothing to worry about, and I want to believe it.

This is difficult to do because, of course, there is no such thing as 'normal'. Health is entirely individual; what is cause for concern in one person means nothing for another. I am fortunate, or not, that because of my past diagnoses and bulging medical file everything I report is investigated extremely thoroughly. For example, I once mentioned to a podiatrist that I sometimes had pins and needles on the bottom of my big toes, and three months later I was sitting in front of an eminent neurologist at a specialist hospital, staring at his politely baffled face as I tried to explain why I was there, an enormous stack of blood test results on the desk in between us. The gears of the UK's National Health Service (NHS) grind slowly but inexorably, and sometimes it feels like I'm on a treadmill that I don't control. I am lucky, so lucky, to exist in a system that spits out appointment letters but no bills whenever I express a concern. It feels extremely stupid to say that I sometimes wish I was taken less seriously, that doctors were more inclined to 'wait and see' where I am concerned. I think their solicitude and efficiency give me an extra but unavoidable layer of anxiety about my health: I prevaricate about whether to even ask for help, because I know that it will be offered and I'm terrified of wasting time that could be given to someone more worthy of it. My situation sounds like every hypochondriac's dream, and yet here I am wishing things were different. Perhaps that restlessness, that eternal doubt, is what truly defines this state of mind.

For those who exist in a healthcare system that is not free at the point of use, like the US, the situation is very different. When every visit to a doctor or hospital can result in hundreds of dollars in charges just for attending an appointment, let alone undergoing any testing, treatment or prescriptions, it adds a whole extra layer of stress and complication to the already fraught relationship between hypochondriac and medical expert. The performance anxiety that I feel in trying to accurately represent my symptoms and experiences to a doctor would be amplified many times over with so much money at stake. As the *DSM-5* notes, health anxiety sufferers tend to be split into those who are 'care avoidant' and those who are 'care seeking', and I do wonder how many of the former group avoid the regular reassurance of a visit to the doctor not because they fear it, but because they cannot afford it. Even for those who are seeking a firm diagnosis of a health anxiety or a related disorder, the evidence suggests that the cost of this can be very high, the ill-defined characteristics and blurry boundaries of this condition requiring many appointments and tests to confirm. And this is for those who have full or partial access to health insurance: census data suggests that about eight per cent of the US population, or 27 million Americans, do not have any coverage at all. Hispanic, Indigenous and Black people are far more likely to be uninsured than white people too, further compounding historic marginalisations. This prompts some uncomfortable questions about who has the luxury to be a hypochondriac, a condition so often defined by its contact and interaction with medical care. Those with health anxiety who are cut off from this basic necessity by inequity and injustice have little choice but to suffer alone and in silence.

The hypochondriac, regardless of their situation, never feels like they are standing on solid ground. Medical advice changes all the time as new discoveries are made and best practices are developed. What might have been unremarkable when you were a child is now considered cause to make an emergency appointment. Context matters too: medical probabilities change with age, location, gender and other factors. Experts can disagree too – more than once I have clung to a doctor's assertion that there is nothing to worry about, only to be told by someone else on a different day that there really is cause for concern. For much of the time that I have been working on this book, Covid-19 has dominated the narrative of global health, and that has also altered the constant assessment of what is normal. When I first started reading about the emergence of the virus in China, I started to panic a little about my future panic – a very hypochondriac thought pattern, to be scared of the fear itself – but when cases started rising in my area, I largely found the experience oddly calming. Other hypochondriacs I have spoken to about this confirmed that they experienced this contradictory reaction too. The world's biggest health emergency of the last century and we, the citizens most anxious about health, stare it serenely in the face. Not quite: I developed what I now recognise as some rather extreme coping mechanisms to handle the horror and the uncertainty of those early pandemic months, such as spending hours a day reading statistical appendices about case data and unnecessarily cleaning the packaging of all our food with disinfectant. But what made this different for me and lots of others with similar inclinations was that – at least in the early months – everybody else was doing this too. We were no longer the outliers, with our irrational fears and our imaginary illnesses. That boundary between what is reasonable, justifiable fear and what is hypochondria had suddenly moved. Suddenly, we were *normal*. Even with everything else that was happening, this was immensely comforting. The threats that had previously only been visible to those constantly on heightened alert were now widespread and even sanctioned by health authorities. As Santiago Levín, president of the Association of Argentine Psychiatrists, put it eighteen months into the pandemic: 'Health anxiety in a situation like the one we're living through is normal, appropriate, and expected.'

The experience of the past few years has made me realise that so much of the distress associated with hypochondria is social, born of feeling isolated from and disbelieved by others.

It makes me think of something that I once heard a comedian say as a punchline: 'I have a phobia of things that can kill me.' It got a big laugh, because a phobia is usually defined as an excessive or irrational fear, but really, what could be more rational than fearing things that could harm you? There is, surely, no shame in wanting to stay alive. The words we use to draw the boundaries between what is a reasonable or legitimate level of fear are subjective and flexible: irrational, excessive, indulgent, unreasonable. There is no absolute and immovable point at which sensible precaution becomes irrational fear. It depends on who you are, what you are, where you are. And that malleability makes hypochondria impossible to plan for or predict. It shapes itself around whatever beliefs and circumstances exist in that moment.

I have long felt that the Elizabethan poet John Donne is a peculiarly hypochondriacal writer. Both his poetry and his prose are stuffed with references to illness; sickness is his favourite metaphor for a whole host of different concepts and emotions. He writes constantly of the slow, gradual decline of the mortal body into the grave. In 'Elegy on Mistress Boulstred', he addresses Death directly, personified as a ravenous diner at a cosmic feast at which all of humanity will be served up to him eventually. This demon plays with his food, however, toying with us as we age and decline: 'Now wantonly he spoils, and eats us not, / But breaks off friends, and lets us piecemeal rot.' Only love has the power to withstand mortality, as Donne says in 'The Anniversary':

> When thou and I first one another saw:
> All other things to their destruction draw,
> Only our love hath no decay;

Donne's poetry is stuffed with surprising ideas and phrases, making it impossible to not come across something startling every time you read it. In 'An Anatomy of the World', for instance, he devastatingly deconstructs the notion that there is any such thing as 'being well':

> There is no health; physicians say that we
> At best enjoy but a neutrality.
> And can there be worse sickness than to know
> That we are never well, nor can be so?

His prose work *Devotions Upon Emergent Occasions, and severall steps in my Sicknes* – in which the famous phrase 'no man is an island' appeared – is a foundational text of hypochondria. Written while Donne was in the grip of a fever that left him physically incapacitated but entirely conscious, *Devotions* has become something of a staple in the small world of hypochondria criticism. It is barely permissible to publish anything on this topic without mentioning it. And why wouldn't we? It is a magnificent literary achievement that was written 400 years ago yet still provides one of the freshest and, to my mind, most accurate accounts of what it is like to be sick with a disease you cannot name.

Donne was taken ill in November 1623 with what is thought to have been a relapsing fever. He believed it to be a reflection of his internal sinfulness and that he was dying; of course, he documented his thoughts and feelings throughout in a series of twenty-three meditations upon his condition. They have titles like 'The patient takes his bed' and 'They warn me of the fearful danger of relapsing'. It is part sickbed diary, part medical record, part devotional text. In between his prayers to God and accounts of purging treatments, he muses upon the intertwined nature of health and mortality. All health is an illusion, he laments, and no matter how hard we work to maintain it, it can be taken from us in a mere moment:

> We study health, and we deliberate upon our meats, and drink, and air, and exercises, and we hew and we polish every stone that goes to that building; and so our health is a long and a regular work: but in a minute a cannon batters all, overthrows all, demolishes all; a sickness unprevented for all our diligence, unsuspected for all our curiosity; nay, undeserved, if we consider only disorder, summons us, seizes us, possesses us, destroys us in an instant.

At the end of the work, feeling better, he nonetheless turns his mind to the ever-present possibility of the fever's sudden return. It is all the more fearful, he says, because it remains unknown:

> Upon a sickness, which as yet appears not, we can scarce fix a fear, because we know not what to fear; but as fear is the busiest and irksomest affection, so is a relapse.

Devotions appeared extraordinarily quickly. It was first published in January 1624, just weeks after Donne's convalescence. As both a near-contemporaneous record of his illness and the culmination of a lifetime of writing about sickness and death, it is unsurpassed.

However, not everybody agrees that Donne's evident and lifelong preoccupation with all the ways in which a human body can malfunction is evidence of a hypochondriacal mind. The critic Elaine Scarry argues that Donne's 'astonishing alertness to disease' is 'not only intelligible but inevitable in the context of the intimate details of his day-by-day life'. Put simply, the context of Donne's life means that it was not unreasonable for him to fear sickness and see its possibility in every new day, therefore he cannot be said to be a hypochondriac. It is certainly true that Donne, even by the standards of the period in which he lived, experienced great trauma and loss. By the time he was nine years old, his father and three of his sisters had died. His stepfather, John Syminges, was a doctor and young John grew up around his bloody, visceral practice at St Bartholomew's Hospital in the City of London. When Donne was sixteen, Syminges also died, and then when he was twenty-one his brother Henry died horribly in prison of bubonic plague after being arrested for allegedly sheltering a Catholic priest, and Donne did not dare visit him in case he contracted the plague too. He was married to his beloved wife Ann for sixteen years, during which time she was pregnant twelve times, from which they had ten living children, three of whom then died before they reached ten years old. Another daughter, Lucy, passed away when she was eighteen. At various points, he refers to his house full of children as 'a hospital' and once grimly joked that at least when a baby died, there was one fewer mouth to feed, but one did have to find the burial expenses. Ann also died a few days after giving birth for the twelfth time, leaving Donne to spend the last twenty-five years of his life alone, working and worrying about the waves of sickness that were constantly passing through the city.

Against such a backdrop of tragedy, it seems inevitable and almost sensible that Donne would be preoccupied with sickness and mortality. Weighing the evidence rationally, he might well have concluded that his health could fail any moment, or another child be taken from him. In such a situation, is it not reasonable to be afraid, and to experience those fears not just in the mind but in the body too? That said, the fervour of Donne's despair in *Devotions* does not indicate a measured response to early modern death rates. He is wild and passionate, indicating that the knowledge illness can strike at any time is as disabling as the illness itself.

> O multiplied misery! we die, and cannot enjoy death, because we die in this torment of sickness; we are tormented with sickness, and cannot stay till the torment come, but pre-apprehensions and presages prophesy those torments which induce that death before either come ... O perplexed discomposition, O riddling distemper, O miserable condition of man!

In the eighteenth of the twenty-three meditations that make up *Devotions*, he visualises his soul being released from his body and moving towards 'everlasting rest, and joy, and glory', but after only one step, it pauses, missing its former 'dwelling-house'. Even when contemplating the divine, Donne clings to earthly, bodily existence. Being homesick for the body that you are still in feels to me like the very essence of hypochondria.

Donne is revered now primarily as a poet who merged the romantic and the spiritual. His extravagant, transgressive imagery – 'It sucked me first, and now sucks thee, / And in this flea our two bloods mingled be' – is what transfixes the modern reader. The potency of his preoccupation with sickness and death has been subsumed into this, as he says in the opening of 'The Canonization': 'For God's sake hold your tongue, and let me love, / Or chide my palsy, or my gout', his eloquence on the matter of health interpreted as yet another way in which he understood the true meaning of life: to love and be loved.

And yet, it was when he was writing about his own experience of illness, in *Devotions*, that Donne put the most of himself upon the page. Indeed, he visualised his own body cut up and arranged for readers to peruse:

> They have seen me and heard me, arraigned me in these fetters and received the evidence, have cut up mine own anatomy, dissected myself, and they are gone to read upon me.

At the same time as Donne was feverishly transforming himself into text, another writer was engaged in a very similar project – albeit one that would see him more overtly associated with worries about health and sickness. First published in 1621, Robert Burton's *The Anatomy of Melancholy* marks a crucial moment in the history of hypochondria. The full subtitle is indicative of its capacious ambitions: 'The Anatomy of Melancholy, What it is: With all the Kinds, Causes, Symptomes, Prognostickes, and Several Cures of it. In Three Maine Partitions with their several Sections, Members, and Subsections. Philosophically, Medicinally, Historically, Opened and Cut Up'. Although melancholy had begun as a humoral term, Galen of Pergamon had enlarged on the original Hippocratic observations of melancholy to add that sufferers often exhibited 'bizarre and fixed ideas'. He wrote in *On the Affected Parts* that 'there are patients who think to have become a sort of snail so that they must escape everyone in order to avoid having their skull crushed'. By the seventeenth century, melancholy had come to be used as a catchall for the many and diverse types of mental distress that people experienced. Anxiety, sadness, pensiveness, introversion, grief, phobias, delusions and more all came under this heading, as did the physical symptoms associated with this type of humoral imbalance, like rashes, abdominal pain and difficulties sleeping. In fact melancholy is, by Burton's account, an intensely physical experience:

> There is almost no part of the body, which being distempered, doth not cause this malady, as [it involves] the brain and his parts, heart, liver, spleen, stomach, matrix or womb, pylorus, mirach, mesentery, hypochondries, mesaraic veins ...

Melancholy had 'infinite varieties,' Burton said, and 'scarce two of two thousand concur in the same symptoms. The tower of Babel never yielded such confusion of tongues, as the chaos of melancholy doth variety of symptoms.' Reading Burton, one comes away with the dizzying feeling that melancholy is everything and everything is melancholy. It is simply the condition of existing in the world. Just like melancholy, hypochondria, or 'splenetic hypochondriacal wind', was rife, if Burton is to be believed. It is 'a disease so grievous, so common ... than to prescribe means how to prevent and cure so universal a malady, an epidemical disease, that so often, so much crucifies the body and mind'. As a subset of the broader – vaguer – idea of melancholy, hypochondria incorporates many of its features, with the added reference to the specific parts of the abdomen called 'hypochondries', where a painful spleen or liver sits. Alongside its physical elements, he writes too of the 'fear and sorrow' that plague those with this affliction. There is a hint, too, that the imaginary component that would later come to dominate is already present. Hypochondria is already reaching out beyond the rational, the possible. Some sufferers, Burton writes, 'will not be persuaded but that he hath a serpent in his guts, a viper, another frogs'. The sensations they feel are too strange to be explained just by the habitual contents of the body. Only by introducing an incongruous amphibian will they make sense.

Melancholy, by the time Burton came to write about it, was acquiring associations with the way technological advances were changing the world. Information overload was a concern in the seventeenth century, as it is today: people were worried about there being too much information available now that printed books were easily accessible and the effect that all this text might have on mind and mood, for instance. Burton himself owned an extraordinarily large number of books – over 1,700, a collection no doubt funded in part by the success of the *Anatomy* during his lifetime. The fact that Burton's idiosyncratic project enjoyed such popularity speaks to the widespread fascination with the strange ways in which the mind could malfunction. At the same time as Renaissance Europe was captivated by the glass delusion and the men who believed they were breakable, melancholy had become 'achingly fashionable'. Only those of a brilliantly creative and sensitive temperament were thought to experience the condition, and the furrowed brow and isolated sorrowfulness of the sufferer became the very latest in trendy affectation. It was also a mark of class and wealth, since those without means were unlikely to be able to afford a doctor to endorse their melancholic diagnosis – a factor that will only become more important in centuries to come, as we delve into the idea of who is afforded the luxury of being a hypochondriac. Hypochondria as we understand it today is the successor condition of this form of melancholy, with all of its shape-shifting symptoms and vain fixation on the fragility of the self.

*

The *Anatomy* has compelled and baffled readers for 400 years, in part because it straddles the divide between the age of superstition and the age of reason. This is a book that looks backwards and forwards from a crucial point in the evolution of thought about the body and the mind. Even the title represents this – 'anatomy' during Burton's lifetime meant 'analysis' or 'logical dissection', but was also beginning to be associated with the practice of dissecting the human body to advance knowledge of it. Although the book is presented as a medical textbook, it is far more eclectic than that. It is an encyclopaedic work of over a thousand pages, which Burton revised and expanded five times before his death in 1640. Every single page is littered with classical quotations, most of them densely woven into Burton's own meandering prose. It is the last book of its kind, representing the tail end of the doctrine of 'general learning', which assumed that any one scholar could master all of the major disciplines of learning. Burton's address to the reader at the start of the book contains the first known use of the term 'polymath' in the English language, and perhaps you need to be one yourself to fully understand everything that he writes about. And yet it is a revered text, beloved of writers and medical historians alike. Some of the works from which Burton quoted are now lost to us, so it is a vital source of thought about melancholy and human suffering through the ages. Byron called it 'the most amusing and instructive medley of quotations and classical anecdotes I ever perused', but not everybody found it such easy or pleasant reading. Samuel Johnson's biographer James Boswell – himself a sufferer of this hypochondriacal melancholy who even wrote a column under the pseudonym 'the Hypochondriack' – recorded in his *Life of Dr Johnson* that 'Burton's *Anatomy of Melancholy* was the only book that ever took him out of bed two hours sooner than he wished to rise.'

In biographical terms, Burton was a direct contemporary of the physician William Harvey – they were born just a few months apart in 1577 and 1578 – and the latter's groundbreaking work on the circulation of the blood first appeared only a handful of years after the first edition of Burton's magnum opus. Another significant step forward in medicine came twenty years after Burton's death in 1640 when the Royal Society was founded in London, formalising a burgeoning interest in empiricism and the scientific method. Very little of this progress is visible in the *Anatomy*, though. Burton's understanding of the human body is still heavily invested in the humours. The book is full of references to people suffering melancholic symptoms, which are affected by 'celestial influences', because of their ingrained temperament or because of the influence of elements that are 'hot or cold, natural, unnatural, innate or adventitious, intended or remitted, simple or mixed, their diverse mixtures and several adustions, combinations'. In spite of the more esoteric elements, more recent scholars have praised Burton for his intuitive understanding of human psychology; one named him the 'scholarly and humanistic precursor of Freud' and said that the range of his interests, as far as 'the facts of human behaviour are concerned, was identical to that of our great modern analyst of the psyche'. According to the philosopher Jennifer Radden, many of the foundational tenets of today's mental health treatments can be found in Burton. His emphasis on the power of the imagination to shape a sense of agency corresponds with the theory of cognitive behavioural therapy, she argues. He also insists on a good preventative regime of bodily health – what we might today call 'self-care' – and praises the therapeutic power of music as 'a sovereign remedy against despair and melancholy'.

Burton was, of course, speaking from experience as he was

afflicted with the very condition that he had devoted his life to dissecting. 'I write of melancholy, by being busy to avoid melancholy,' he says. I wonder how well this worked: did spending decades dwelling on the precise nature of the sadness that engulfed him help him to eliminate it? I don't know if keeping busy by contemplating the infinite variety of your own problems would be recommended by a therapist today. This is the secret joke of the whole of the *Anatomy*, which Burton hints at in his preface. He addresses the reader directly, warning against becoming too immersed in the symptoms of melancholy, in case they start to affect you:

> Yet one caution let me give by the way to my present, or
> my future reader, who is actually melancholy, that he read
> not the symptoms or prognostics in this following tract, lest
> by applying that which he reads to himself, aggravating,
> appropriating things generally spoken, to his own person
> (as melancholy men for the most part do) he trouble or hurt
> himself, and get in conclusion more harm than good.

This has the ring of something learned by bitter experience. Burton had received his own diagnosis of melancholy as a young man, when he travelled from Oxford to London to consult the renowned physician and astrologer Simon Forman. At the time, Burton was suffering from the classical presentation of hypochondriacal melancholy, with a 'general malaise' accompanied by stomach complaints. Forman's horoscope not only reveals his propensity towards melancholy, but also predicts the year of his death. He will live until 1640 – when he will have attained the age of sixty-three – and then pass away suddenly from an unknown cause. Burton set much store by astrology, as the *Anatomy* demonstrates, and took this prediction very much to heart. It seems to have provided him with a sense of certainty that was otherwise lacking amid the thousands of pages of material he had accumulated about why someone might be experiencing both mental distress and physical symptoms. He wrote his own epitaph for his memorial in Christ Church cathedral and made sure that the astrological chart was included next to the moulded image of his own likeness. His death matched the prediction so perfectly that rumours abounded that he had taken matters into his own hands in order to prove correct the horoscope by which he had lived his life. A seventeenth-century Oxford chronicler, Anthony à Wood, wrote that 'several of the students did not forbear to whisper among themselves, that rather than there should be a mistake in the calculation, he sent up his soul to heaven through a slip about his neck'. This was just gossip though – had there been a serious suggestion of suicide, Burton would not have been buried with honours on hallowed ground. Already, the balance of certainty had shifted, and those left behind after Burton's death were unwilling to believe that an astrological prediction could have come true. Hypochondria, too, was in motion. Soon, Burton's view of the condition would be supplanted. But one legacy of his writing which still endures is the connection between hypochondria and an awkward kind of humour.

Taking his lead from the humours, Burton speaks of 'hypochondriacal or windy melancholy'. The symptoms of this complaint are ambiguous and a matter of some medical dissent, but he lists some common indicators, including 'continual wind about their hypochondries' as well as 'sharp belchings, fulsome crudities, heat in the bowels, wind and rumbling in the guts, vehement gripings, pain in the belly and stomach'. More than four centuries ago, then, hypochondria was already a very farty state of being. And farts are inherently funny, as much as we might pretend otherwise once we have reached adulthood. I still remember fondly the day my sister and I discovered among the DVD extras for the 2003 festive romantic comedy *Love Actually* a scene in which a child character is reprimanded by his stern headmistress for writing that his 'Christmas wish' is for people's farts to be visible like little soap bubbles in the air. A sequence follows imagining how this might work: grandma farting at the Christmas dinner table, unable to blame the dog; a choir member farting during a service, with the whole congregation turning to stare at them; the queen farting while walking the corgis with her family. The boy's mother pretends to share the teacher's embarrassment but once out in the corridor applauds him for creating a 'top-quality gag'. Director Richard Curtis introduces the clip by saying that is one of the elements cut for the final edit that he most mourns, and I couldn't agree more. The romantic elements of that film have largely not aged well in the past two decades, but the farting scene is a timeless piece of comedy.

We laugh about the bubble farts for the same reason that we do about hypochondria: because what is meant to be private and unseen is made public and visible. In the society and culture in which I was brought up, nudity and bodily functions are something to be hidden away. Unless there is a very good reason, such as old age or serious (real!) illness, we are expected to control and conceal regular everyday acts like menstruating and passing waste. Hypochondria overrides this instinct to bodily secrecy, though. The drive to find answers for our worries sees us asking embarrassing questions of our friends or sends us to medical clinics, willing to bare all if it will result in an explanation. The same taboo that makes jokes about bathroom malfunctions and digestive accidents funny works here as well. Hypochondriacs just seem too interested in the scatological, and what else can we do but laugh at them for it.

But as well as this obvious bodily humour, hypochondria is funny in the way that any kind of delusion can be funny. Torturous and unrelenting as it can be, it is also amusing. Hypochondriacs behave neurotically in their distress, checking and rechecking the same body parts while asking absurd questions like 'do my veins look more blue than usual?' or 'do you think my toes might have shrunk?' They obsess over bodily fluids and functions and submit to invasive medical investigations in a way that can read to others as ludicrous, even farcical. And they often compulsively share the ridiculousness of their thought patterns with those around them, always seeking reassurance. As with all the best types of humour, there is an edge of cruelty to this too. For centuries, people have been laughing at those who see things that aren't there – partly because it is comic to see someone clutching at thin air and partly as a defence mechanism against something they don't understand – and imaginary illnesses are just as ripe for this treatment. The humour is a form of self-defence, though: the one cracking the joke is invested in the unlikelihood of the hypochondriac's illness being real. It is presumed that they are mistaken, and thus fair game for mockery. Doctors joke about hypochondriacs too – or at least they used to, before recent efforts to destigmatise mental health conditions began. They used to call them 'crocks', 'turkeys', 'cranks' or 'gomers', the last one being a slang acronym for what they wish they could really say, 'get out of my emergency room'. As an added incentive to normalise this kind of humour, the hypochondriac is, to an extent, in on the joke and aware of how their behaviour is perceived. This is one of the most singular features of this state of mind; I *know* I am being silly about this mole or that itch,

but I persist in it anyway. And it is in that self-knowledge that
the comic potential resides. You can't make any jokes about me
that I haven't already heard inside my own head. Although that
doesn't mean that they don't sting.

We can laugh at hypochondria because the fear seems outlandish, the tragic outcome unlikely. For those who don't live
with a brain constantly knotted in doubt about their state of
health, it is amusing to see a fit, outwardly healthy-looking
person take on the role of an invalid with no discernible
cause, just as it is funny in the most basic sense to see a virile
young comedian do an impression of a fussy old man. Any
kind of unreasonable or out-of-character behaviour can elicit
this response – see the many, many stand-up routines about
road rage – but there is an added frisson to matters of health
because it is already so performative. I can only tell if you are
well because of a few subjective visual cues and because you
tell me that you are. Without being aware of it, we constantly
act out how we feel inside for the consumption of others, but
how they react to this information is beyond our control.

The most blackly comic experience I have ever had with a
healthcare provider occurred over a long weekend in my late
twenties. It began when I was on the train, being whisked
through a tunnel under London at a rattling, clanking speed,
sitting in a deserted carriage in early evening. The glass panes
in the doors at either end were lowered so that a strong wind
was blowing through the train as it surged forward into the
darkness. The lights flickered off for a moment and when they
came back on, it felt like I was watching a scene from a film. I
see the breeze pick up my hair from where it lies in its usual
lank straight lengths on my shoulders and blow it away from
the direction of the train's destination – a familiar sensation

from travelling in a fast car with the window down. Except that strands of my hair are lifting entirely away from my head and, as I watch, being tossed up into the middle of the carriage by the air's flow. They dance there for a moment on the current of air that is piercing the train. My hair had always been dark and fine, but when it had grown back years ago after my second round of chemotherapy, it was even darker and finer. These almost black strands seem to writhe under the harsh strip lighting in the ceiling, like cells under a microscope, before spiralling away down the carriage, through the open window at the end, and on through the rest of the train. My mind goes with them for a moment, imagining them shooting out into the still, dark tunnel behind and then gradually floating from side to side, like an autumn leaf just released by a tree, until they are swallowed up by the ground.

Despite the panic that followed, I remained aware that healthy people don't suddenly lose chunks of hair while travelling on public transport. When I got to my destination, where I was supposed to see a play with a friend, I was too unsettled to contemplate sitting in a darkened theatre for several hours, unable to check whether I had covered the auditorium's carpet with loose hair. I made my friend sit in the theatre bar with me instead and insisted that she talked about anything else to distract me while I drank a lot of water. On the way home I took the bus – less of a brisk, hair-destroying breeze – and did a lot of reading online about what constitutes the normal range of hair 'fall'. Around fifty to a hundred strands a day is usual, I learned, and most people don't even notice its going. My fingers itched with the effort it took not to touch my head and see how much more wanted to come out. The major causes of sudden hair loss are stress and an underlying illness, which seemed to me like the perfect one-two punch to set anxiety spiralling. I probably had a serious illness and now I was stressed about it; no wonder this was happening.

Two days later, late on Sunday when the options for appropriate medical advice were limited, I finally decided that I couldn't last any longer without help. I called the NHS's non-emergency helpline and tried to put my best case forward that I needed assistance. I didn't make it further than the standard triage questions at the start of the call, though, because I unthinkingly answered 'yes' when asked 'are you currently bleeding?' The person on the other end of the line was not a medical professional, but rather a phone operator who was patiently transcribing my words into a computer system that then told him what to ask me next, and as soon as he registered my positive response to this question alarms started going off. He was instantly directed to follow a new script that aimed to help me stem the blood loss while the computer automatically dispatched paramedics to my location. His voice suddenly grew intense and urgent, switching from the studied neutrality that had characterised his initial manner to a higher gear that seemed to say 'now this is a *real* problem'. It was only with great difficulty that I managed to make him, and the computer, understand that I was only menstruating and not haemorrhaging in a way that would require hospitalisation, urgent surgery and a transfusion. Once I had got him to call the ambulances off and I was sure that there were no sirens currently heading my way, I couldn't face trying to explain why pulling out handfuls of hair felt like a serious emergency to me. I hung up and lay back on the sofa, crying with laughter at the idea that I had just narrowly missed having to explain to paramedics that they were here to deal with my period and a handful of loose hair. What had a few minutes ago seemed like an unbearable problem was now far less acute. I somehow felt like I could see myself from the outside and appreciate how ridiculous I was.

I was not cured, though. I would like it to be noted that my hair did carry on falling out for a few days before the rate gradually slowed and I was able to let the problem recede into the background. I did see a doctor about it, several times, and the conclusion was that it was a stress response to something I was never able to define. It has happened several times since, and I do still worry about it, but if my hypochondria is a jukebox with many different songs that can be played, let's just say that this one isn't in heavy rotation these days.

Of the roles that we all play at some point in life, the hypochondriac is the most naturally satirical. In a certain cynical light, it reads as a parody of genuine sickness, albeit an unconscious one, an exaggerated caricature of something that ought to be utterly authentic and sincere. In the period between the classical followers of Hippocrates and the Early Modern renaissance of melancholy, there developed a moral dimension to the unhappy collision of mental bleakness and physical weakness: to become too consumed by one's melancholy, to allow the black bile to become burnt and overpowering, was to commit the sin of acedia. This word is derived from the Greek word ἀκηδία, literally meaning 'non-caring state', and was interpreted by medieval Christianity to mean a lethal state of listlessness, in which the sufferer was heedless even of the duty they owed to God. The guilt, blame and shame that so often accompany hypochondria now, I think, has some roots in this sinful form of melancholy.

Nobody blurred the boundaries between genuine sickness, comic performance and hypochondria more deftly than the French playwright and actor Molière, who was born about the same time that *The Anatomy of Melancholy* was first published. Molière, the stage name of Jean-Baptiste Poquelin, began his career aspiring to be a great writer and interpreter of tragedy, but the quirks of fate and royal patronage made him a purveyor of comedy and *opéra bouffe* instead. It is fitting, though, that the subject matter at the heart of his final play *Le Malade imaginaire* is dark and sombre. Strip away the farcical action and the musical interludes, and you have a deeply sad drama about Argan, the 'imaginary invalid' of the title, who is consumed by the fear that he is seriously ill. This terror taints all aspects of his life, making him irritable and supremely selfish. He self-medicates with a vast array of quack remedies, some of which make him feel worse and send him further into the dismal recesses of his troubled mind. His every decision is underpinned by this mortal anxiety about his health. The main focus of the plot is his attempt to marry his daughter off to a doctor, against her wishes, so that he will always have a medical attendant close by. A sacrifice of sorts: her life for his life. He is the hypochondriac pushed to extremes, with no character traits left that have not been transformed by his fears.

Of course, because this is French comedy from 1673, many aspects of Argan's condition and treatments are played for laughs. One of the bevy of doctors that flock around him is 'Monsieur Purgon', who has a seemingly endless array of laxatives that will purge any known complaint from the body – with plenty of windy, digestive gags to really drive the point home to the audience. Molière's biographers have speculated that when it came to writing about Argan's symptoms and his endless dissatisfaction with the medical profession, the playwright was drawing on his own experiences. We know that Molière suffered from ill health for much of his adult life, with weak lungs and a chronic cough that became so frequent in the early 1670s that he wrote it into the script as a persistent trait

for Argan – an act of heartbreaking practicality that seems to
merge writer, actor and character together into a single figure
of suffering. The diagnosis of tuberculosis has been suggested
latterly, which seems to fit the symptoms he recorded, and the
fact that his condition was much better during the years in
which his troupe were perpetually on tour and they spent the
winter years in the warmer climate of southern France, away
from the damp, smoky chill of Paris.

Molière's decline accelerated when his troupe began to enjoy
the favour of Louis XIV and moved permanently to play at a
theatre within the palace built for Cardinal Richelieu in the
heart of the city. The cold, damp conditions coupled with the
sheer volume of work he was doing wore upon him, until he
reached the point where he either had to incorporate his symptoms into the plays he was not only writing but acting in, or
remove himself from the stage entirely. We can track Molière's
preoccupation with his health through his work. He had written
plays satirising the medical profession before: 1665's *L'Amour
médecin*, for instance, features five doctors who were based on
real-life Parisian physicians, each with their own idiosyncrasy
mercilessly magnified by the playwright. One is obsessed with
vomiting and talks of nothing but emetics, another is fixated
on bloodletting, a third cannot speak without elongating every
syllable interminably, and so on. They quarrel constantly
over every diagnosis, but are united in their reverence for the
Hippocratic method, believing that following precisely in the
footsteps of the Ancient Greeks is far more important than
ensuring a patient's comfort or recovery. It's a clever double
parody: Molière is caricaturing these specific practitioners, but
also the system within which they practice. It's the work of an
intelligent, anxious writer laden down with his frustrations and
fears about his health, who has received no meaningful help

from the supposed experts he has consulted. He can't stop coughing up blood, and all they want to do is open up his veins to let more out and make him throw up whatever is left inside of him. There is nothing to do apart from make people laugh at it, and by extension, him.

In the final act of *Le Malade imaginaire*, Argan pretends to have succumbed to his many maladies so that he can see how his family and friends react to his death. I imagine Molière had followed his character down this route in his mind already, wondering how his actress wife, the company, his many doctors and his demanding patrons would take it when the cough finally took control of him. For such a prolific and public figure, very little record remains of Molière's life outside the theatre if he even had one, which on the strength of the surviving evidence seems unlikely. His marriage is a case in point: at the age of forty he wed seventeen-year-old Armande Béjart, the sister or possibly the daughter of his long-time friend and business partner, the actress Madeleine Béjart. The couple were not well matched if the hostile pamphlets poking fun at their infelicity are to be believed. She flirted with other men, and he was jealous. Despite 'separating' after the birth of their daughter in 1665, they continued to work together in the theatre constantly, often acting as husband and wife on stage, like a bickering couple from a farce brought to life. Armande both played and defined major roles in many of her husband's works in the 1660s and 1670s: she was the star of *La Princesse d'Élide*, Elmire in *Tartuffe*, Lucile in *Le Bourgeois gentilhomme* and Angélique in *Le Malade imaginaire*. Her crowning achievement was also his: her acclaimed performance as Célimène in his masterpiece *Le Misanthrope*, her talent showcased in the role of a flirtatious young wife obsessed with social climbing that was written both for her and about her.

No record survives of the barbs that the playwright and

leading lady flung at each other during rehearsals or while waiting in the wings for a performance to begin, but in the gap my
mind writes in exchanges that mirror their onstage dialogue.
Threats shouted, heads tossed, doors slammed. Their marriage
was over outside the theatre, but that barely seems to have
mattered since Molière scarcely existed anywhere else. He was
fiercely productive, appearing on stage as the comic lead in play
after play at night and spending his days dealing with publishers, agents and managers. In the fourteen years that he led his
troupe at the Théâtre du Palais-Royal, they put on ninety-five
different plays, of which he authored thirty-one. Somehow,
during this time he and Armande had three children, two of
whom died in their infancy. More tragedy to weigh on the mind
of a sick man. Hypochondria, especially the kind rooted in a
misunderstood or misdiagnosed condition, brings mortality
very close, its wings just brushing the side of your face. In *Le
Malade imaginaire*, the hypochondriac's 'death' is played for
laughs, with Argan's wife overjoyed that she can now claim her
inheritance, while his daughter is distraught with grief. And of
course, because this is a comedy, Argan gets to leap up again
and reveal that it has all been a joke, a performance. Do the
audience notice that he is still coughing into his sleeve, even
as they laugh at his post-death antics?

In the final scene, Argan declares that he will himself
become a doctor: surely no disease would dare kill off a
member of this vaunted profession? And he can become one
that very night without years of study: Argan's brother knows
of a place that will confer this honour upon him straight away,
no questions asked, like a quickie wedding performed by an
Elvis impersonator. The play ends with a musical interlude in
which dancers surround Argan in celebration of his elevation
to the best-worst profession. All is well.

Until isn't. On the day of *Le Malade imaginaire*'s fourth performance on 17 February 1673, Molière was coughing more than usual. He refused to cancel the performance, or to let another actor go on as Argan, no doubt thinking of the gossip and scandal that would result in Parisian theatre-going circles if the famous playwright was seen to have abandoned the cast of his own play so early in its run. He doggedly acted through the pain, disguising his coughs as Argan's coughs, but at the climactic moment where the imaginary invalid claims the title of doctor for the first time, encircled by an absurd, dancing and singing chorus of other surgeons, he was 'seized with a convulsion'. Was it Argan or was it Molière who doubled over, coughing and shaking, unable to draw a clear breath? The audience couldn't be sure. The playwright had so success-fully written his fears and his symptoms into the character that the usual outcry and concern at an actor being taken ill onstage never occurred. I was once at a West End production of *Hamlet* when an actor was taken seriously ill on stage, and something similar happened: for what felt like a very long and silent moment, nobody either in the audience or on the stage was sure if it was King Claudius who had staggered and fallen or the person playing him. Then the director leapt from the wings to catch him and the spell was broken; we all realised we had been sitting motionless while somebody was suffering. The curtain came down and an ambulance was called. In the same way, Molière's performance is difficult to disentangle: a very sick man was pretending to be a healthy man who imagined that he was mortally ill. Hypochondria is not a case of a healthy person pretending to be sick. The hypochondriac truly believes themselves to be unwell, and may in fact be so. Should you believe them? The boundaries are utterly blurred.

Molière made it to the end of the play without breaking

character fully, but began shivering and coughing again as soon as it was over. His young protégé, the actor and upcoming playwright Michel Baron, arranged for his mentor to be carried to his nearby residence in a sedan chair and put to bed there. Soon, Molière began coughing up blood again and sent Baron to summon his wife. By the time she arrived, Molière was dead, having choked on his own blood.

The hypochondriac remains a stock character in comedy to this day. In the 1960s, the downbeat, naturalistic English comedian Tony Hancock played up the self-involved, absurd figure with quips like 'Hypochondria is the only illness I don't have.' Later, Woody Allen's neurotic hypochondriac characters in films like 1986's *Hannah and Her Sisters* cemented many of the familiar tropes. Allen plays a whiny, emasculated character who, the viewer is made to understand, is constantly taking himself to the doctor with imaginary conditions that amount to nothing. Then the latest in this long line of consultations actually turns up something: slight hearing loss, accompanied by dizziness and a ringing sound in his ears. He undergoes a montaged battery of medical tests, an experience that culminates in a weekend spent in utter paranoia while waiting for the final appointment when all will be revealed. We see him, red-eyed and panicking, sitting in the doctor's office as the doctor enters and his scans are hung up for viewing; we hear the specialist say the dreaded words, 'I'm afraid the news is not good. If I can show you exactly where the tumour is and why we feel that surgery would be of no use . . .'. The camera zooms in on Allen's face as he clutches his hair, paralysed by fear, muttering about how he is going to face eternity 'not later but now'. Then the frame moves again: the doctor walks into the room for a second time, hangs up the scans and says 'you're just fine'. The first consultation was a hallucination, a hypochondriac's delusion. It was all in his head after all, but the effect of showing both outcomes in one long, rolling scene like this is to, briefly, include the viewer in the horror of forever being trapped between the two possibilities. After receiving the good news, Allen's character enjoys about five seconds of dancing down the street to exuberant big-band music before the utter meaninglessness of existence crashes down on him once more. He isn't dying today, but what about tomorrow?

Seinfeld is the obvious inheritor of the comic hypochondriac, with the character of George Costanza periodically bothering his friends with his persistent fears that he has whatever illness he recently saw covered on television. In the thirteenth episode, 'The Heart Attack', George's hypochondria gets star billing, after he suffers what he thinks is a heart attack while eating a salad, having watched a show called 'Coronary Country' the night before. He has all the symptoms – 'Tightness ... Shortness of breath ... Radiating waves of pain!' – but his friends keep eating and cracking jokes, unconcerned. This time, surely, will be like all the other times. When George does make it to the hospital, Jerry intercepts the doctor and receives the good news that there was indeed no heart attack before George hears it, so that he can then torment his panicking friend by staking a pre-emptive claim to prized possessions after he dies. In a twenty-two minute episode, George manages to hit all of the major hypochondriac tropes. Having been hospitalised, he then visits a (much cheaper) holistic healer, and is finally actually injured in an ambulance crash on the way back to the hospital after ingesting a noxious quack remedy.

It isn't just on screen that hypochondriac humour has thrived. The long-time cartoon editor of the *New Yorker*, Bob

Mankoff, once described hypochondria as 'my faithful muse' and the inspiration for a large segment of his work. Some of his best are the one-frame 'pocket' style cartoons, in which a single scene is depicted with a short caption. The setup of doctor or therapist and their patient is instantly recognisable, and when accompanied with a line like 'Well, Bob, it looks like a paper cut, but just to be sure let's do lots of tests,' or 'But if you cure my hypochondria I won't have any hobbies' the cartoon makes it clear that this is not a serious consultation, but one that the viewer is permitted, even encouraged, to laugh at.

This vein of pop culture continues into the twenty-first century, with animated sitcoms like *Family Guy* and *South Park* featuring hypochondriac characters. In the 'Bloody Mary' episode of the latter from 2005, we even got a comedic take on my own panicked visits to the office bathroom mirror to check for lumps, with the character of Randy standing there to rail against the world after attending an Alcoholics Anonymous meeting and leaving convinced that he has a terrible disease. 'It's not fair, why did you give *me* this disease?' he howls, heavenwards, while shaving his head. In the next scene, he is in a wheelchair and looks the complete invalid, while still drinking, and is telling his son that 'this disease is just eating me up'.

Plenty of stand-up comics still have routines about their hypochondria; some build entire touring shows around it. Unlike other material with a long pedigree, it still seems to get the laughs. Marc Maron has a line in his special *End Times Fun* that announces, explains and ridicules his own history with the condition in one breath: 'My father was a doctor, which means I was a hypochondriac. How else are you going to get their attention?' He has been doing this bit for over a decade, too, in shows with titles like *Thinky Pain*. In April 2020, he described himself as a 'recovered hypochondriac' and explained that it was realising the fundamentally absurd nature of what he was doing that finally helped to pull him out of this state of being. He was a college student at the time and constantly preoccupied with his fear that he had prostate cancer – a highly unlikely diagnosis at his stage of life. Suddenly, while standing in a bedroom as a urologist friend of his father's inspected his penis, Maron had a clarifying moment and realised that everything about the situation was 'ridiculous'. Noticing the absurdity of it allowed him to move past it. I only wish that my run-in with the emergency services over my hair loss incident had given me the same kind of lasting clarity.

In using this story as a staple of his shows, Maron is drawing on a long-established association between hypochondria and comedy in Jewish humour. This is a tradition built on self-deprecation and irony. There are many, many high-profile examples of this – the work of Woody Allen, Jerry Seinfeld, Lenny Bruce, Freddie Roman and others speaks for itself – but nobody is sure exactly why hypochondria came to be such a strongly Jewish theme. It permeates literature too, via Philip Roth's alter ego Nathan Zuckerman, who shares some of the writer's own obsessive personality traits and is a hypochondriac obsessed with his own mortality. In her memoir about their troubled relationship, Roth's second wife Claire Bloom writes extensively about the author's health anxieties and some alarming episodes he experienced, including once suddenly losing the ability to breathe while swimming alone in a pool, which he survived by clinging tenaciously to the edge to keep his head above water until it passed. Later, he checked himself into Silver Hill, a psychiatric hospital in Connecticut, and explained in a statement that this decision was in part due to anxiety about his health and in part because of disappointment at the poor reception of his 1993 novel *Operation Shylock*. Once their marriage had irreparably broken down the following year, Bloom recorded that the only communications she received from her soon-to-be ex-husband that did not include a furious covering letter were to do with their health insurance paperwork, indicating its starring role in his mental priorities. 'He seemed to be on closer terms with my insurance plan than with me,' she recalled.

There is no hard evidence that Jewish people experience a higher incidence of anxiety of any kind, yet this remarkably persistent stereotype of the neurotic, health-obsessed Jew survives. 'It is hard to distinguish epidemiology from anti-Semitism,' one expert points out. Centuries of persecution seems like reasonable grounds to fear for your safety and your health, but there is more to it than that, one therapist has suggested. Intergenerational trauma, often denied or overlooked, needs an outlet, and joking about hypochondria is a way of drawing attention to this in a relatively safe way. Another theory suggests that the nature of Jewish scripture and observance embeds the habit of constant examination and analysis, which then gets turned inwards. Precariousness breeds uncertainty for any group, and as the philosopher Simon Rawidowicz lays out in his 1948 essay 'The Ever-Dying People,' many generations of Jewish people have had ample reason to believe that their generation will be the last.

Each always saw before it the abyss ready to swallow it up. There was scarcely a generation that while toiling, falling, and rising, again being uprooted and striking new roots, was not filled with the deepest anxiety lest it be fated to stand at the grave of the nation, to be buried in it.

Hypochondria is funny, and it is also not funny at all. The fact that we laugh is an expression of cruelty, prejudice and, at best, insecurity. Mortality is uncomfortable. To take the hypochondriac seriously would be to acknowledge that we are all always standing much closer to the edge than we realise.

4

Spirits, Vapours and Nerves

The strangest aspect of my teenage medical adventures concerns the preventative fertility procedure I underwent just before my nineteenth birthday. The cancer treatment that was planned for the rest of my year was of such an advanced level of toxicity that it had a high chance of affecting my future fertility – or, as it was explained to me, the drugs could nuke my ovaries. Therefore, it was strongly recommended that I had eggs extracted beforehand, so that in the future it would 'give me options'. I was mostly detached from the process, being a student with no interest in parenthood who was far more concerned with her own survival than any hypothetical future children, but the word 'options' was repeated enough times that I agreed to take part.

As a result, I spent a few months hanging around in waiting rooms with women at least a decade older than me who were also having to inject themselves with hormones daily. They took me under their wing, the strangely anomalous teenager in the fertility clinic. We compared our bruised stomachs and swapped tips for when the plastic applicators broke and exposed the needle points. This was an education worth having; just their stray comments and half-whispered conversations taught me more about women's health than any amount of official classes at school had, as well as the disregard with which it is treated. Everybody had a horror story to share in the most casual way: I heard tales of intrauterine devices that had fallen out suddenly during work presentations, of months spent hopped up on hormones, of round after round of in vitro fertilisation (IVF) that had failed for no discernible reason. At every turn, there had been a doctor who disregarded their wishes or ignored what they had to say.

After a month of hormone injections and near-daily ultrasounds, my ovaries were deemed to have expanded to a sufficient size that the extraction could take place. If anyone explained to me in detail what this would involve beforehand, I have no memory of that conversation. Dressed in a hospital gown, I was taken into what looked like a conference room at the clinic and put on a trolley. A kind of twilight sedation was administered, so that I was woozy and partially numb in the relevant area but otherwise fully conscious of what was happening. A medical team wielding an ultrasound probe and a large needle got to work. A thick tube leading away from me and through a hatch in the wall to a laboratory bulged and throbbed ominously as the extracted material was sent away to be frozen. It hurt, a lot.

Afterwards, my father drove me back to my university accommodation. We shared a takeaway before he had to leave. I obediently followed the advice I had been given to get some rest and take paracetamol if I felt any discomfort. After having my insides repeatedly pierced by a large needle, I'm not sure how there could be any other outcome. I don't remember thinking it was strange at the time that I wasn't given any other pain relief options. Years later, when I observed the elaborate after-care arrangements and prescriptions involved in an ingrown toenail operation, I began to wonder if perhaps not all pain was treated equally.

In 1885, after her daughter Katharine was born, the writer Charlotte Perkins Gilman experienced what she called 'the breakdown'. Now identified as a period of postpartum depression, she described in her autobiography how the then new condition of 'nervous prostration' was attracting derisive reactions. 'To be recognisably ill one must be confined to one's bed, and preferably in pain,' she wrote. 'That a heretofore markedly vigorous young woman, with every comfort about her, should collapse in this lamentable manner was inexplicable.' All of the exhortations she received from family and friends to 'use your will' and 'get up and do something' achieved no improvement, and five months after Katharine was born, Charlotte weaned her so that she could go away for a restorative trip to California – the doctor's suggestion. It worked, temporarily. A month after she returned, she was 'as low as ever', struggling with respiratory problems and facing the demoralising idea that she was 'well while away and sick while at home'. A famous nerve specialist was called, who turned out to have his own preconceived ideas about her family, the Beechers, which included such members as the suffragist Isabella Beecher Hooker and the author Harriet Beecher Stowe. ' "I've had two women of your blood here already," he told me scornfully.' The diagnosis? Hysteria.

The journey of hypochondria up the body, from being tangibly rooted in the liver and abdomen to today's understanding of it residing in the brain, is not a smooth one. And beginning in the late seventeenth century, this condition made a protracted diversion via the womb, a much-theorised organ with its own vast literature and conflicting history. The century or so in which the womb stars in hypochondria's story marks a chaotic and fascinating chapter in this tale. And to understand how that came to be, we have to go back to when the womb was known by the Greek word *hystera*.

Hysteria, as the conditions associated with the womb had come to be known by the time of Hippocrates in the fifth century BCE, is a complex web of shifting afflictions that has supported entire biographies of its own. Like hypochondria, it is present in the very earliest surviving records – as we saw earlier, the Ancient Egyptians were writing in the Kahun Papyrus more than a thousand years before Hippocrates about their cures for 'terrors of the womb' that move around the body causing problems. By the time the Greeks were considering the womb, its vitality and mobility had become a matter of much dispute. In the *Timaeus*, Plato describes the womb as 'the animal within', which if not allowed to fulfil its purpose of creating children, 'gets discontented and angry' and wanders about the body causing mischief. The second century CE medical writer Aretaeus further characterised it as 'like some animal inside an animal', almost a separate being of its own within the human body, with its own motivations and priorities. Galen, however, is more circumspect in his appraisal of this theory, demonstrating that it was far from universally accepted. The image, though, of the womb as a kind of manacled beast within a woman's body has been extremely influential. Whether it moves or not, this questionable organ became associated with behaviour that is 'voracious, predatory, appetitive, unstable' and thus indicative of female frailty and instability.

It was in 1667 that hysteria and hypochondria collided. Thomas Willis, physician and founding member of the Royal

Society, published a groundbreaking work on the brain and set off a whole new direction for hypochondria. When it was translated from Latin into English in 1681, this tome had the not at all catchy title of *An Essay of the Pathology of the Brain and Nervous Stock in which Convulsive Diseases are Treated of.* In it, he drew on both his academic research and his medical practice to pull together an impressive picture of what we would now call the nervous system. In a radical departure from centuries of medical tradition, Willis put the brain at the centre of all human illness, although he also refers frequently to the swelling of the hypochondria when speaking of the abdomen. The crucial section for our story, though, concerns a patient of about forty years old, to whom Willis was summoned in his capacity as one of the most popular and consulted doctors in London.

This man suffered with sporadic periods of incapacitating convulsions and vertigo, which both patient and doctor could feel spreading 'from the bottom of his belly upwards, towards his heart and breast, and from thence to his head'. Initially Willis believed him to be in 'more need of Exorcisms, than of Medicines' – an echo of the religious and spiritual conceptions of such symptoms in centuries past – but after observing several sequences of convulsions and the way in which the patient was able to sense that they were coming hours or even days ahead of time, the doctor came to a different conclusion. The symptoms were attributable 'to the evill affections of the brain, and nervous stock,' he decided, and the cause of the problem 'did lie in the head itself', rather than in any external force or abdominal malfunction. If this affliction had presented in a woman, he continues, it would have been called hysterical and blamed on the womb. The fact that it was being experienced by somebody without a womb, therefore, was further evidence that these hysteria-like symptoms came from elsewhere in the body. Men could have hysteria too, he was suggesting, although that term didn't quite fit, given that it was a specific reference to the womb, the *hystera*. More than that, Willis was advancing a new understanding of the interaction between body and disease that was coalescing at this time. The Hippocratic tradition, still widely adhered to in large part, was founded on the belief that disease came from within the body, caused by the imbalances that were present. This notion was now being superseded by its inverse: that diseases were external, classifiable entities that affected most bodies in a similar way. While the history and state of a particular patient's body did have an impact on how a disease manifested, it was only in the relationship between these internal and external factors that the true nature of an illness could be discerned.

This came to fruition in the work of Thomas Sydenham, sometimes called 'the English Hippocrates'. In his 1682 *Epistolary Dissertation*, he compared the symptoms of what were supposedly two distinct and anatomically rooted conditions – hysteria and hypochondria. Women were more likely to develop the former, while men generally experienced the latter, but the two were indistinguishable, he argued. 'Hypochondriasis ... is as like [hysteria], as one egg is to another,' he wrote. Others were coming to the same conclusion: the seventeenth-century German chemist and philosopher Georg Ernst Stahl stated that 'there is no essential difference between these two affections'. They were just two gendered variations on the same theme. Women had hysteria and men had hypochondria. This was both an expression of the general direction of medical thought and a reflection of the inequalities baked into the way that patients were diagnosed and treated.

The explanations given for why hysteria and hypochondria were connected were varied and, at times, contradictory. Some, like Sydenham and Willis, were inclined to separate both conditions from their anatomical roots and cite the brain as a common point of origin – and since everybody had a brain, this explained the similarities across all patients. Others, like Stahl, preferred to find mirroring physical symptoms that showed how the two conditions manifested differently in men and women. This had been happening for a while; back in 1609 an apothecary named Henry Joly published a treatise that combined hypochondriacal and hysterical diagnoses, associating the negative effects of the organs of the hypochondrium with that of the womb. This soon became a fleshed out system of its own: hysteria was rooted in the womb and hypochondria in the liver and spleen. Women expelled excess blood with intense and irregular menstruation while men did the same via vomiting or haemorrhoids. Both experienced gastric distress because their wandering abdominal organs interfered with the smooth operation of the stomach and intestines. This more classical and physical understanding of what some experts have called 'hysteria-hypochondriasis' did not survive long, though. The majority movement in medical research was towards the brain and associated systems and away from purely physical explanations for conditions that were primarily experienced in the mind. The previous understanding of the body was shattering and something new was reforming.

By the time Willis was working on the brain, though, hysteria and the adjective 'hysterical' were already so gendered that men could not possibly be described by these words, so a new term – hypochondria – had to be co-opted to explain the similarities. The theorists were well aware of this gendering, and indeed it added to hysteria's hypochondriacal appeal. 'Among the diseases of women, hysterical affection is of such bad repute that ... it must bear the faults of numerous other affections,'

Willis wrote. Hysteria was too easy to blame, he went on. If a woman presented with 'disease of unknown nature and hidden origin', her doctor was highly likely to 'blame the bad influence of the uterus' rather than look for any more specific cause. The patient would be left alone with just that baggy, vague label of 'hysteria' and little or no treatment options. Rather than providing any kind of cure, it's easy to see how this would lead to fears about all the possible illnesses lurking in the body that were not being attended to properly because the presence of hysteria had been declared. Being diagnosed as a hysteric at this time would make my anxiety about my health worse, I think, rather than better.

So it proved for Charlotte Perkins Gilman. Her eminent nerve specialist's treatment regimen for hysteria was modelled on the principle that the patient needed absolute rest – from thought itself, it seems. She was told: 'Live as domestic a life as possible. Have your child with you all the time . . . Lie down an hour after each meal. Have but two hours' intellectual life a day. And never touch pen, brush or pencil as long as you live.' She was to be completely isolated from family and friends, to eat a fatty, rich diet and to remain in bed at all times. She was forbidden even to feed herself. Months of rigidly following this programme sent Gilman into a state of 'mental torment' that resulted in her making babies out of rags and trying to hide from 'the grinding pressure of that profound distress' by crawling into cupboards and under beds. Eventually, in 1887, she and her husband agreed to end their marriage. Very, very gradually, her exhaustion abated and her ability to read and write returned, although she never reached her previous capacity again. 'That leaves twenty-seven years, a little lifetime in itself, taken out, between twenty-four and sixty-six, which I have lost,' she later reflected. Her nerve specialist had not believed her when she said that she needed intellectual stimulation to feel like herself, and she lived with the consequences of his 'domestic' prescription, delivered at such a vulnerable moment, for the rest of her life. I think there is a tendency today, in this overstimulated age of burnout and ceaseless corporate exploitation, to think fondly of the rest cures and convalescent homes of past eras. We think of endless days with nothing to do but nap and stare at the ceiling while kind nurses in vintage costumes bring regular delicious meals. Gilman's experiences should stand as a warning against this fantasy. She wrote later that her supposed rest cure put her 'so near the borderline of utter mental ruin that I could see over' and that she only began to recover when she abandoned its restrictive, isolated rules entirely. Sometimes emptying your mind is the worst possible thing that you can do.

In 1888, at the age of twenty-eight, Gilman returned to work out of financial necessity and in 1892 published a short story that was heavily inspired by her experience of hysteria and its treatment. 'The Yellow Wallpaper' became a classic of American feminist fiction. It is written as a series of journal entries by a nameless female protagonist, who is spending a summer in a large country house with her doctor husband. She tells us at the outset that she has been unwell with a 'temporary nervous depression, a slight hysterical tendency'. To cure her, her husband locks her in the top floor of the house and forbids her to undertake any kind of mental or intellectual work at all. The bed is screwed to the floor and she is watched perpetually by her suspicious sister-in-law. She begins to think that the sickly yellow wallpaper in her room is mutating and moving, and that there is a woman crawling on all fours trapped inside it. Early on in the story, she records the powerlessness of her situation:

> You see, he does not believe I am sick! And what can one do? If a physician of high standing, and one's own husband, assures friends and relatives that there is really nothing the matter with one but temporary nervous depression – a slight hysterical tendency – what is one to do?

Her husband and her brother, also a doctor, have absolute control over her mind and body. She cannot escape the room with the yellow wallpaper and gradually she becomes the crawling woman trapped inside.

When I seek help for a health problem, whether real or imagined, I take the risk that I will not be believed. So do many, many others. The evidence is all around us. Studies have repeatedly shown that the perception of pain is subjective, and that women, non-white people and other marginalised groups are routinely given lower pain scores than the 'default man' so beloved of medical research. Heart disease kills twice as many women in the UK as breast cancer, yet the former is still often viewed as a 'man's illness' and the warning signs that make it into public awareness campaigns are not applicable to women's bodies. Serious and painful health conditions that only affect women, like endometriosis, regularly go undiagnosed for years as the symptoms of sufferers are dismissed and they are fobbed off with platitudes. People experiencing conditions like myalgic encephalomyelitis, chronic fatigue syndrome and long Covid that may have myriad intermittent symptoms for which there is no complete medical test can struggle for months or years to find an expert who will take them seriously. Disabled and overweight people have difficulty getting their illnesses considered as anything other than additional symptoms of their existing bodies. The maternal mortality rate for Black women is shockingly high compared to their white counterparts: in the UK they are four times as likely to die in childbirth and 2.6 times as likely in the US. The perception that these patients experience lower levels of pain or more frequently 'time waste' with invisible symptoms discourages people from seeking help, further compounding the inequalities. This is the hidden horror of hypochondria: even when someone has a real and pressing medical problem, its taint can still touch them, making it more likely that they will be dismissed without the assistance they need. Every time a hypochondriac goes unheard and untreated, it solidifies the idea that some people are unconsciously making it all up and that they don't need help.

Throughout my explorations of hypochondria's twists and turns through medical history, I have been struck by how often the examples I find concern women's health, from the gynaecological case studies in the Kahun Papyrus of Ancient Egypt to the young woman from Thasus with the 'melancholic turn of mind, from some accidental cause of sorrow' who appears in the Hippocratic Corpus. Where there is doubt, there is hypochondria, and it so often seems to be women whose symptoms go unexplained.

For an otherwise healthy, privileged woman, the discovery of fertility problems is often her first encounter with health anxiety. There is so little certainty, so little control, to be had in the process of IVF that very few come through it with their mental state unaffected. Because I was so young when my eggs were extracted, I was granted an exemption to the standard rules for cancer-related IVF. Usually, the NHS funds ten years of egg storage for patients in my situation, but I received fifteen years in acknowledgement of the fact that twenty-eight years old is still young to know whether you want to have a family or not. Thus, a decade and a half after my treatment, I crept into a toilet cubicle at my office to take the phone call from the fertility clinic and had to tell a doctor whether I wanted my eggs destroyed or if I would be paying to keep them in their subzero limbo from now on.

As it happened, the voice on the other end of the line belonged to one of the doctors who had treated me originally, and she remembered me – it wasn't every day that she did egg retrievals for teenagers, she explained. She was extremely kind, asking how I had been and whether I had indeed become a writer as I had said I wanted to when I was in her consulting room at the age of eighteen. I kept spinning out this small talk, postponing the question that I knew had to be asked. I screwed up my courage. Was there any way of telling if I needed the frozen eggs, I hesitantly inquired. Taking on the storage fees was a major financial commitment and it would be nice not to have to budget for that. I had been told that my chemotherapy had a more than fifty per cent chance of destroying my fertility, but no follow-up testing had ever been done to discover if that was the case. The response from the doctor was far from reassuring. No, she said, there was no test she could do to definitively answer that question. If I wanted to have children, I should start trying to conceive and, if it worked, we would know that everything was fine. If it didn't . . . Well, that sentence was left hanging.

As I left my twenties behind, the conversations about IVF that were going on around me among friends and colleagues became increasingly jaded and frustrated. Even in the UK, where some treatments are funded by the NHS, people end up paying thousands of pounds out of pocket for their treatment, and in the US this is the default experience. One and then another woman I knew received an unsatisfying verdict of 'unexplained infertility' after many failed attempts. Another was told 'As far as we can see, this should be working, but it isn't.' Hypochondria thrives in the absence of better information. Is it any wonder, given all of the prejudice that lies in our past, that women end up asking themselves: *is it my fault?*

The demise of the humours as the dominant explanation for why the human body behaved the way that it did left a gap in understanding. For thousands of years, ideas about balance, fluidity and circulation had been held by these metaphorical liquids. Phlegm, blood, black bile and yellow bile had formed a language of their own and given the body a unified voice that physicians and laypeople alike could understand. Without them, alternative theories became a cacophony that it is hard to make sense of. The interest in hypochondria and associated conditions intensified just as the settled explanation for it was disrupted, and this caused an explosion of new ideas about how the body worked, how the mind was connected to it, and what it all meant for human existence. Treatises were published at a great rate from the 1670s onwards, and a new confusing and contradictory vocabulary appeared as people groped towards a fresh way of understanding what they felt and why. This 'mumbo jumbo', as one historian terms it, brings us to yet another phase in hypochondria's existence: utter chaos.

This is where the overlapping, multidirectional nature of hypochondria's story is most acutely present. The primacy of humoral theory was declining, but this was not happening in tandem with the rise of a unified replacement. As we saw with the collision of hypochondria and hysteria, physicians, philosophers and theorists were simultaneously disproving what had gone before while also borrowing from it. Different people were arriving at the same new concepts by completely antithetical routes. Parallel theories ran alongside each other during this time, with different schools of thought barely comprehending each other. Hypochondria, for all its mysterious dimensions, had been a settled thing, defined by its connection to a specific area of the body and to black bile and melancholy. Without this explanation, it became a jumble of misunderstood symptoms in desperate want of a system that made it intelligble. It had been like the single stream of a river, twisting and turning along the variations of the humours, which then hit an insurmountable obstacle with the advent of the Enlightenment and the burgeoning anatomical understanding of the human body. The stream split around the barrier, fracturing into multiple channels of thought that were all attempting to reach the same eventual destination. To those floating down one of these rivulets, it might have seemed as if they were in what would soon emerge as the main river again, but from our vantage point today, this criss-crossing delta of ideas is wild and bewildering and entirely lacking in purpose. And to understand what hypochondria was soon to become, we have to sample them all.

The first explanation that emerged from this chaotic period when hypochondria was a condition of either the mind or the body, or both, or neither, was something called 'animal spirits'. Conceived of as some kind of bodily fluid, sometimes literal, sometimes figurative, these 'spirits' had been mentioned in medical literature since the time of Ancient Rome. The followers of Galen, whose work dominated European, North African and Middle Eastern scholarship for over a thousand years after his death in the second century CE, believed that animal spirits were produced in the brain and functioned as a link between the body and soul. They moved around the body as messengers and, according to the theory, interacted with the humours, which could impede or change the activity of the spirits via their imbalance. If the humours became too hot or corrupted, for instance, the animal spirits might become more heated too, causing the person to behave out of character – to become more passionate or impetuous, in line with beliefs about how overheating humours caused a hotter temper. In a healthy, even-tempered person, the spirits should be distributed evenly around the body, but when a moment of high passion occurs, they collect dangerously in certain areas – the face, or the limbs in a situation that requires violence or a rapid escape. The spirits could even play a role in moral decision-making, pushing the person they inhabited towards good or evil.

Exactly what animal spirits were made of is impossible to say. Like the humoral fluids – black bile, yellow bile, phlegm, blood – this new substance was figurative in nature. Nobody in the centuries after Galen counted on being able to pierce the skin and capture some in a vial for analysis – such an idea would have been laughable. The spirits existed to explain the link between mind and body, rather than as an actual liquid you might expect to be able to wet your finger with. And yet at the same time physicians and patients alike believed implicitly in their actual presence in the body. This there-and-not-there sensibility is hard to reconcile now, in our age of empiricism and insistence on evidence and verification. For a medical concept, it begins to feel uncomfortably spiritual, like something born of faith rather than science.

The meaning of the phrase animal spirits – or *spiritus animales* as they were more likely to be called in the medical treatises of the sixteenth and seventeenth centuries – was entirely flexible. They were therefore the perfect vessel for new ideas about sensation and disease once the humours began to decline in popularity; they were redefined and repurposed as required. Thomas Sydenham channelled his concerns about the imbalance of the relationship between mind and body into them, and made them extremely influential in his concept of health, even while admitting that he didn't really know what they were. It is in his work, too, that the animal spirits are explicitly linked to hypochondria – it is in 'the irregularity of the spirits' from which the lack of harmony between mind and body so often observed in those suffering from this condition stems. The animal spirits dominate these two realms, the mental and the physical, and any inconsistency in their quantity or quality spells trouble. Quite what one was supposed to do about this, though, is unclear. Everybody agreed that a deficiency in animal spirits was a bad thing, and likely to lead to complex and hard-to-treat conditions like hypochondria and hysteria, but there was a huge variation in understanding exactly what this pesky fluid might be.

Everything about the body feels in flux at this time. A few decades before Sydenham was grappling with the question of what is mind and what is body, the physician William Harvey published the provocative theory that blood circulated in the body, pumped by the heart, rather than being formed in the digestive system and then absorbed by the tissues of the other organs, as per the humoral tradition. 'I began privately to think that it might rather have a certain movement, as it were, in a circle,' he wrote in 1628's *De Motu Cordis*, feeling his way cautiously towards one of the most significant scientific discoveries of the millennium. The idea of circulation rippled through all other aspects of medical inquiry. The likes of René Descartes and, later, the Dutch anatomist Herman Boerhaave were already beginning to think about the body in a more mechanical and less holistically spiritual way, and Harvey's theory pushed them even further. What if the body contained more than one circulatory system, and in it the brain played a similar part to the heart? In this newly hydraulic view of the body, the brain was a gland secreting a liquid – animal spirits – that then flowed through a system of tubes to every organ and limb. There had to be something that explained both the intangible connection of body and mind, and conditions like hypochondria that resulted from a disordered relationship between the two.

Harvey's work was based on the dissection and observation of both humans and animals, and several scholars tried to apply this empirical approach to the circulation of animal spirits, or 'nervous fluid' as some began to call it. Unfortunately, the results were inconclusive: some microscope work seemed to show evidence of hollow 'nerves' through which the spirits could pass, like a plant's capillary, while other investigators claimed to have seen only solid fibres that contained no liquid. Diverging explanations appeared: perhaps these refined vessels of sensibility were too tiny to be seen by the human eye even when assisted by the most powerful of lenses, or perhaps they were solid but acted like silken threads, with moisture adhering along the fibres like water on a string. Descartes imagined a system of solid fibres or 'bell ropes' that were connected to valves which controlled the flow of gaseous animal spirits around the body. A stimulus in the arm would trigger a valve in the brain that would direct the spirits to the right place to create sensation and reaction.

As the move towards a more practical and anatomical understanding of the human body progressed, the questions became more tangible and specific. How were these fibres produced? What were they made of? What happened if there were too many in any one place in the body? Their operation was discussed in the language of engineering: the spirits were said to be boiling or condensing, flowing or seeping. Tension was highly significant and became linked with different moods and temperaments. Elasticity suggested a healthy equilibrium, while lax, flabby or weak fibres indicated a constitutional tendency towards hypochondria. A smooth flow of animal spirits around the body was considered vital for an accurate perception of health. Crucially, spirit disorders were expressed as mental conditions – an early hint that these chaotically overlapping theories and systems were leading towards a new paradigm in which illness was not only a function of the physical body. If the spirits were chaotic and disturbed, the patient would likely suffer from madness or mania, while if they were insufficient and sluggish, the person was probably hypochondriacal. After over a thousand years of discussion and inquiry it was still no clearer what animal spirits actually were, but by the early eighteenth century it was agreed that not having enough of them could make you believe in illnesses that weren't really there.

The notion of circulation remained very important, even as the doctrine of balance that underpinned humoral theory diminished in significance. It seems as if it has always been difficult for us to picture the human body as a solid mass of meat; something must always be moving inside it. And this is how we arrive at 'vapours', the second of our three hypochondriacal possibilities from this era, which from the late seventeenth century gained currency as the agents of mysterious malignity in the body. Defining exactly what a vapour was thought to be is tricky – the word, usually spelled 'vapor' without the usual additional 'u' common in British English now – describes both the substance that moved around the body and the condition that it caused. Vapours were a kind of exhalation, or a fume, a movement of particles in gaseous form (before this concept was understood) that were released by certain organs akin to the way that mist rises from the ground on a cold morning. When I try to picture a vapour, I think of woodsmoke rising from a clearing and up through the trees, filtering between the leaves on its way towards the sky. The transparent glass vessel that is the body slowly fills with it, clouding the surface and hiding the interior from view. There are no tubes or vessels to direct the vapour; it flows and expands to fill the available space, moving in directions that have no visible cause. Smoke and steam have long been used in Indigenous cultures to send messages to beings in both this world and others; within the body, vapours were thought to carry information and sensation from one part to another.

It is an arresting image, this corporeal entity filled with purposeful air, although not an especially logical one. We can trace its origins back to the early seventeenth century. In what is generally considered to be the first text in English about hysteria, Edward Jorden's 1603 book *A Briefe Discourse of a Disease Called the Suffocation of the Mother*, the condition is attributed in part to the spread of a noxious substance called 'vapors' around the body from the afflicted womb – once again the problem is connected to the dysfunctional female body. The physicians of Ancient Rome and the Arabic scholars of the Middle Ages likewise worried about airy substances emanating from the womb – the idea that blood or semen could be retained by the uterus and then putrefy there, producing a rotten stench that invaded the rest of the body and caused illness, was a pervasive one. Jorden's vapours are similar, but don't have such a clear point of origin, or a link to a recognisable external process like decomposition. They are merely there, a convenient way for Jorden to move away from the idea of a 'wandering womb' and still explain how a condition like hysteria that was rooted in the organ could be having an effect in the head and heart. As the title of his book suggests, hysteria was sometimes known at this point as 'the suffocation of the mother' – an evocative and horrible name, but in fact a step towards rationality, since this identified it as a 'natural disease'; symptoms that had previously been ascribed to witchcraft and the devil were now thought to have a biological cause. The vapours rose invisibly up through the body, suffocating the patient and producing their most common symptoms: a feeling of unease, sudden violent spasms and the sensation of continual choking in the throat, even though there was no discernible obstruction. The breathing apparatus was particularly affected, with the diaphragm and lungs clogged with vapours so that the infected person could neither inhale nor exhale. It wasn't just the womb that produced vapours, either. The apothecary Henry Joly identified vapours arising from the spleen and liver, hinting at a vaporous dimension to the hypochondriac region of the abdomen too.

A hundred years later, the relationship between vapours and what we now understand to be hypochondria was cemented by another English physician. John Purcell published *A Treatise of Vapours or Hysterick Fits* in 1707, and defined this new bodily mechanism thus: 'Vapours ... is a distemper which more generally afflicts humankind than any other whatsoever; and Proteus-like, transforms itself into the Shape and Representation of almost all Diseases.' This chameleon-like capacity to mimic other illnesses and the difficulty of isolating vapours as the cause of anything did not prevent Purcell from writing hundreds of pages on the subject. Reading his descriptions now, it is impossible to regard his version of the vapours as anything other than what we would call generalised health anxiety: the symptoms can be anything at all, and there is very

little that a physician can do about them. Vapours were especially dangerous during the first moments of sleep, when 'the
vapors which rise in the body and ascend to the head are many,
turbulent, and dense. They are so dark that they waken no
image in the brain; they merely agitate, in their chaotic dance,
the nerves and the muscles,' according to the Italian physician
Paul Zacchias. Vapours were strongly associated with mental
disturbance and a loss of bodily control, as well as unexplained
instances of physical malfunction like choking or skin discoloration. But there were plenty who dissented from the murky
power of the vapours: even as Purcell was laying down the law
on the subject, French physician Martin Lange was despairing
of this whole avenue of medical thought, describing vapours as
'one of these vague words to which no distinct idea has been
attached, & used by physicians to cover their ignorance, or to
amuse the People with words'. This instability and uncertainty
left a residue that survived long after the vapours themselves
had evaporated.

Thomas Willis, pre-empting the third influential theory of
mind, body and sensation, thought that animal spirits existed
alongside something he called 'bodily nerves'. Thanks to his
work dissecting human brains, he was able to posit a connection
between the brain stem, these fibrous 'nerves', the fluid that he
observed in the spine and the movement of muscles. He even
coined the word 'neurologie' to describe this new field of study.

Willis also found no difference in 'nerves' between men
and women, further reducing the gender-related associations
between hysteria and hypochondria. These fibres were, in
one sense, more observable – the dissection of animal bodies
certainly revealed their presence. George Cheyne, author of
the popular eighteenth-century treatise on nervous disorders

The English Malady, theorised that the whole human body was in fact composed of these thread-like fibres, of which nerves were just one subcategory. These were highly sensitive and transmitted sensation around the body – thus, someone with overactive nerves was more likely to fall prey to the common symptoms of hypochondria. But, like the other two solutions posited for this troublesome crossover point between mind and body, 'nerves' soon came to have a symbolic, as well as a literal, function. The tautness or slackness of one's nerves came to stand in for certain characteristics and behaviours, just as the humours had provided the tendencies towards hot anger or cold melancholy. And this imagery persists to this day: we speak of someone who is 'tightly wound' or 'highly strung' to denote an excess of nervous energy.

Of course, of these three different ways of understanding the connection between mind and body, it was nerves that won out in the end. In 1653, William Harvey was describing the nervous system in a way that chimes with our understanding of it today. 'The nerves are like plantings of the brain, and provide ready intelligence for the organs of sensation; like the fingers of the hand; wherefore the brain neither sees or hears, yet knows all things,' he wrote. Rather than being hollow tubes through which spirits travelled or strings that could be tightened or loosened, nerves were finally understood as a sensory instrument that transmitted information about the body back to the centre of cognition and understanding, the brain. Advancements in anatomy and the study of electricity in the late eighteenth century, building on Willis's work on 'neurologie', eventually provided the scientific backing for what had, for centuries, been just one of several competing theories.

But when I am standing in front of the mirror, checking for traces of whatever ailment is currently troubling me, those displaced explanations for how the interior of the body functions still feel present within me. The hyperawareness of every thread from which I am woven, the feeling of all my strings being wound far too tightly, the fog of fear that spreads through every limb – these are real to me, even if I know they are not real. There is an intense physicality to this, something that the term 'anxiety' alone cannot encompass. Our modern habit of locating this distress entirely in the mind, our focus on mental health, isn't sufficient for all that I feel. The old-fashioned phrases – having a fit of the vapours, having a conniption, suffering with my nerves – give us something that has been lost from the modern terminology. An acknowledgement of the body and all its strangeness.

I once heard the comedian Tiffany Haddish talk about a self-esteem exercise that she had done at a particularly low point in her life, when she was living in her car and performing stand-up for free at clubs. It involved looking at your reflection in the mirror for five minutes, really making eye contact, and saying aloud that you love and approve of yourself. 'The first time I did it, girl, I cried so hard I couldn't even see my own eyes,' she said. She kept doing it, crying every time, until eventually she could bear the sight of her own eyeballs without weeping. I think about this a lot when I see my scared self in the mirror, this other person inside the glass, her body just like my body. Untangling the story of hypochondria has made me appreciate what I have right there in front of me, to be able to look at it steadily, without fear. Our bodies are so strange and improbable. I am such a miraculous jumble of complex systems and processes. What can I do but marvel at the infinite wonder of it?

5

The Rise and Rise of the Quack

How many hypochondriacs are there? This question has many answers. The percentage of the population formally diagnosed with the *DSM-5*'s newly coined 'illness anxiety disorder' is small, a fraction of one per cent, and those with debilitating somatic symptom disorder is even lower. Experts over the past couple of decades have tended to put the rate of general hypochondria somewhat higher, between four and seven per cent. The presence of severe and persistent health anxieties in patients with a serious pre-existing condition is much higher, in excess of ten per cent. One study from 2011 that examined a sample of patients attending hospital clinics in the UK found that one in five had shown clear evidence of health anxiety, while another from ten years before revealed that the proportion of symptoms displayed by patients at two London hospitals that lacked any medical explanation was fifty per cent. With the difficulties in recognising and diagnosing hypochondria, all of this data must be considered approximate. Many more people than this will have known sporadic and unexplained anxiety around their health, perhaps when a loved one is unwell or at a time of particular stress in another area of their life, but never sought medical attention for it. In an entirely anecdotal fashion, I have gathered my own impressions: over the years that I have been working on this book, whenever I tell someone about the subject they will, without fail, either say that they have personally experienced some of what I am describing or that they have a close friend or family member who has. The base rate of hypochondria in the global population is hard to establish, then, but surveys do indicate that it is on the rise. Again, this partial and hard-to-verify information passes the gut check for me: it seems logical in the era of an unfolding pandemic and its consequences that people would register a heightened level of anxiety about illness.

This isn't an effect confined to events since 2020, though. For more than two decades, scholars have been highlighting the incongruity of data around hypochondria and health anxiety: it is far more prevalent in prosperous countries where people have widespread access to advanced healthcare and population-level trends around health and life expectancy are consistently improving. In a much-cited paper from 1988 titled 'The Paradox of Health', Professor A. J. Barsky lays out many of the factors that contribute to this mismatch between the reality and perception of health. More treatable illnesses; a heightened sense of individual agency over wellness via diet, exercise and lifestyle; the growth of a 'giant medical industrial complex'; a mass media that can pull medical data out of proportion; and a general sense that daily life is becoming more 'medicalised' all feature. This, of course, was written long before the internet became a central part of our lives. Now, my search history is the most intimate account of my hypochondria that exists. It is a granular record of every fleeting and near-unconscious fear I have about my health. It's like an involuntary diary, each search term a frozen frame from the whirlwind of my panic. Add to that the economic forces involved, which in places without a comprehensive state-funded healthcare system incentivise rich people to use healthcare as much as possible while depriving the poor of the most basic care, and you have a compelling case for why hypochondria might be described as the marquee condition of our age.

Who has hypochondria is no less difficult a question to answer. The demographic history is just as complex and elusive as that of the condition itself. During the eighteenth century, when the conception of hypochondria was shifting from being a bodily condition to something with a mental component, the image of the hypochondriac was also undergoing a transition: a democratisation. Until then, hypochondria had generally been considered the preserve of the upper echelons of society, and this is certainly the dominant impression given by the cultural records we have.

Hypochondria is a 'disease of civilisation' said George Cheyne in 1733, a consequence of the excesses of an imperial and consumerist society that had abandoned the simplicity of earlier human existence in favour of an indulgent diet and inactive lifestyle. Chronic health problems, especially those that cause ongoing anxiety and require the constant application of medications, were the preserve of the fashionable elite, or 'the Rich, the Lazy, the Luxurious, and the Unactive', as he puts it. Despite their ailments, he makes their existence sound decadent and rather enjoyable: these are people 'who fare daintily and live voluptuously, those who are furnished with the rarest Delicacies, the richest Foods, and the most generous Wines, such as can provoke the Appetites, Senses and Passions in the most exquisite and voluptuous Manner'. That their problems are self-inflicted – 'it is the miserable Man himself that creates his Miseries, and begets his Torture, or, at least, those from whom he has derived his bodily Organs' – does not at all lessen their severity.

The historian George Sebastian Rousseau has shown how, in the mid-eighteenth century, illness was yet another aspect of fashion. The kind of ailments you suffered marked you out as a member of a particular class as clearly as the type of clothes you wore. Only the working classes suffered broken bones or the kind of diseases that were thought to be caused by dirt and degradation: 'If consumption was ... the disease of poverty and deprivation, nerves was the condition of class and standing.' Conditions that came from within, like hypochondria and nervous illness, were associated with refinement, imagination and intellectual activity. The decades from 1750 to 1800 were turbulent politically, with industrialisation rapidly altering the socioeconomic status for thousands and revolutions upending previously entrenched hierarchies. An emerging professional and middle class even began to aspire to the nervous illnesses of the elite as a way to separate themselves from their more humble origins. 'For snobs, parvenus and social climbers, the way to rise was simple: be hyppish, be nervous, be bilious, be rich,' Rousseau explains. Since these posh maladies seemed to have a much lower mortality rate than, say, tuberculosis, the desire to indulge in them is somewhat understandable, given the alternatives experienced lower down the social pecking order.

A hundred years before, Robert Burton was writing enviously in *The Anatomy of Melancholy* of 'common people' in places as far flung as China and America who live 'coarsely' and break all of the Hippocratic rules for diet and lifestyle, but somehow still enjoy wonderful health and long life. 'These men going naked, feeding coarse, live commonly a hundred years, are seldom or never sick; all which diet our physicians forbid,' he says. There is something intrinsic to the 'vulgar' constitution of the poor, Burton thinks – maintaining a sense of difference being vital to maintaining class distinctions, of course – and this is enhanced by the simple lifestyle enforced by poverty. 'Poor people fare coarsely, work hard, go woolward and bare,' he says in a section about 'love-melancholy', before recording that this kind of deprivation is a common prescription for wealthy sufferers.

Wafting among the more sensitive upper classes during this period was also the popular diagnosis of 'vapours'. Louis XIV's physician Antoine d'Aquin regularly reported on his royal master's issues in this area, writing that 'the king has been a victim of vapors for seven or eight years' and explaining that these rose from the spleen, giving the king the characteristic hypochondriac melancholy associated with that area of the body. The vapours transmitted sorrow and a yearning for solitude to the royal head. The ladies at the court of Queen Anne in London similarly suffered, but their doctor was somewhat less understanding – perhaps because of their gender, perhaps because by the early eighteenth century the vapours had come to be so indelibly associated with elusive or imaginary conditions that it was not possible to take them seriously. Upon receiving yet another summons by a princess with indeterminate health problems, Dr John Radcliffe reportedly responded: 'Tell her Royal Highness that her distemper is nothing but vapors. She's in as good a state of health as any woman breathing, only she can't make up her mind to believe it.'

Although the connection between wealth and hypochondria was very visible – and often had a performative element – this is not the whole story. Hypochondria was not only a luxury illness. It was and is still sometimes argued that those living a more precarious existence don't have the time or mental capacity to invent imaginary illnesses to worry about. I have my doubts about this; I suspect that it is a belief at least partly rooted in biased and discriminatory ideas about why the pain of marginalised people matters less, and who gets to record their inner feelings for posterity. For myself, I have found that my worst bouts of anxiety about my health have accompanied periods of life that are unstable for other reasons – times when I am worried about money or uncertain about who or where I want to be. The more content I am, the more luxurious my existence – by which I mean when I am regularly eating vegetables and going outside at least once a day – the less prone I am to the sudden onset of the mysterious pains in my shins or my stomach. Another idea that speaks to this which I have encountered regularly in the academic literature about hypochondria has to do with what is legitimate anxiety and what is unfounded. One theory about why hypochondria proliferates in wealthy societies is purely because we don't consider those contexts to contain many real threats to good health. Someone living in a place and time where unchecked waterborne diseases are a horrifying part of everyday life, however, is not being hypochondriacal in their fear of drinking from the tap; the danger is considered real, not imaginary.

Regardless of how accurate it really is, the story of hypochondria incorporates this class shift in the 1700s. The notion of the condition spreading from the upper and middle classes to working-class people is part of the narrative and a way in which the change from physical disorder to mental state was rationalised. In 1774 Benjamin Rush, an American physician and a soon-to-be signatory to the Declaration of Independence, gave a lecture to the American Philosophical Society in which he compared the medical history of Native peoples in North America with both contemporary American society and other world cultures. He seemed rather proud that hypochondria is now a more democratic condition:

> The hysteric and hypochondriac disorders, once peculiar to the chambers of the great, are now to be found in our kitchens and workshops. All these diseases have been produced by our having deserted the simple diet, and manners, of our ancestors.

On the other side of the Atlantic, James Boswell was coming to a very similar conclusion in his 1778 column 'On Hypochondria'. This condition – which he was prey to himself to such a degree that his pseudonym for his writings in the press was 'the Hypochondriack' – can occur in 'all sorts of men, from the wisest to the most foolish,' he argued. 'I can assure my readers that I have found as dull and as coarse mortals; nay, as silly creatures as ever appeared upon earth, who had all the symptoms of it.'

As new ideas emerged about how the mind and body were connected, hypochondria became untethered from its roots in digestion and luxurious excess, and more associated with mental malfunction. The link between the physical existence of the brain and nervous system with intangible conditions of the mind had a profound influence. No longer did hypochondria belong only to those with the time to indulge in it. Because mental strain was an important component, working-class people were not only capable of contracting it but even more likely to succumb. Socioeconomic changes contributed to this: through the late eighteenth century and early nineteenth century, people were leaving rural communities and moving into rapidly expanding cities, where they worked incredibly long hours in physically demanding industrial jobs while often isolated from extended family networks. If stressful conditions were more likely to trigger latent flaws in the body or mind, then just being working class during the industrial revolution was surely fraught enough to result in plenty of hypochondriacal incidents.

Soon enough, this new kind of hypochondriac began to show up in medical records. Andrew Duncan, a physician at the Edinburgh Royal Infirmary in the second half of the eighteenth century, writes of one hypochondriac he is treating that 'he is a poor indigent man without house or family and to him the accommodations of an hospital are luxurious'. Servants and other types of workers became regular patients – not least because there were beginning to be charitably funded clinics and hospitals that could cater to them. The surviving notebooks of Duncan's students and colleagues in Edinburgh record a number of pertinent cases, along with a sprinkling of desperate imposters who pretend to have mysterious symptoms so they can have a warm bed and some good meals on a hospital ward for a few days. Determining who was a genuine hypochondriac and who was not seems to have been largely a matter of subjective judgement and not a little drama; in one 1780 case a fourteen-year-old boy who claimed to suffer from daily fainting fits miraculously cured himself when the doctor threatened to apply a hot branding iron to his skin. This edge of cruelty in how hypochondriacs were treated at this time, by using shock or violence to jerk them out of their deception or delusion, recalls the tactics used to 'cure' the glass people of previous centuries. The Parisian glassmaker who believed his buttocks were glass was 'fixed' by his physician beating him.

On the official patient roster at the infirmary in Edinburgh was also a fisherman from the Shetland Islands who was admitted with chest pain that sometimes wandered to his abdomen and throat. He also presented some 'windy' symptoms like belching that recall the digestive hypochondria of the past. This collection of maladies was 'altogether the creature of his own brain', his doctor decided, but the 'lonely manner of life and indifferent living' on his remote northern archipelago likely played a part in his condition too. A young miner, John Craig, was also admitted with painful sensations in his abdomen, which sometimes caused him to faint. In his case, the trouble began after a traumatic accident at the coal pit where he worked when his candle went out and he struggled to find his way back to the surface in the total darkness. In other cases, it was observed that hypochondriacal patients were also suffering from malnutrition and seasonal starvation, since they lived mostly on potatoes in winter, when animal products like meat and dairy were scarce. A contradictory picture emerges. Rich people had hypochondria because their food was too rich and their lifestyles too sedentary; poor people also had it because their diets were limited and their work too physically exhausting. A new theory is required to explain this, one that rests not on the conditions a person lives under, or on the impact they had upon the body, but in the person themselves.

In this way, the eighteenth century was a crucial crossing-over point between different social and medical developments and, as such, it offered particularly fertile soil for both quackery and hypochondria to bloom. Up until this point, medical treatment had primarily consisted either of what we might now call lifestyle changes, such as diet or exercise regimes aimed at rebalancing the humours, or 'doctoring', direct interventions or procedures that had to be performed by the doctor to be effective. These might include the application of leeches, the setting of a bone, or the use of a lancet to open a vein for therapeutic bleeding. Such medications that were prescribed existed to support one or both of these primary therapies. But as European society became progressively more consumerist during the eighteenth century, this began to shift. With the rise of manufacturing came the idea that a householder would buy, rather than make, their domestic goods. Especially for those with surplus income, it became more convenient to purchase items ready made that previous generations would have laboured for hours or days to create from scratch. Once people were accustomed to buying everything from cleaning materials to decor, it followed that they also wanted to purchase medicinal items. Good health thus became strongly associated with material goods, with pills and potions taking on the healing properties that had previously been the preserve of a doctor's less tangible advice or operations. In addition, a debate raged among experts as to how much medical knowledge the layperson could be trusted with. Those at the forefront of the Enlightenment's interest in educational liberation – 'enlightenment is man's emergence from his self-imposed immaturity,' Kant declared – argued for the greatest possible spread of medical knowledge so that every person could make informed choices about their own health and be less susceptible to the irrational blandishments of quacks and 'nostrum-mongers'.

In reality, ingesting these pills and potions was unlikely to bring lasting relief, and in fact was likely to make you feel more ill, since the ingredients were often untested at best and highly toxic at worst. With the heightened bodily awareness of the hypochondriac, the changes induced by these 'cures' would send the subject into an even greater level of anxiety, and so the pattern repeated once again. Some quack medications even contained addictive substances like alcohol or opium, ensuring that the patient would most definitely be back for more.

In 1786, a Scottish doctor named John Moore published his medical memoirs, drawing on over thirty years of practice. Within, he charted what we might term 'the hypochondriac's progress' – a sufferer's journey from first contact with a legitimate doctor and then through their descent through the different layers of the medical establishment, official and unofficial, to eventual hopelessness. When this book appeared, hypochondria still had a definite bodily component; Moore uses a footnote to explain that this disease is so called because 'its seat being supposed to be in a part of the belly which physicians call the hypochondriac region'. There were profound mental symptoms, too, though. The patient he described becomes 'particularly watchful of every bodily feeling, the most transient of which he often considers as the harbinger of disease'. This anxiety begins to affect every aspect of life, until he no longer finds enjoyment in anything. Attempts to explain what is distressing him only make things worse:

> To a circumstantial and pathetic history of his complaints, he often receives a careless, and, to him, a cruel answer, importing that they are all imaginary. One who feels a weight of misery more berthensome than acute bodily pain, naturally considers this as the greatest insult.

He consults a 'whole tribe' of doctors, some of whom are able to treat the symptoms of this anxiety, but nothing seems to touch the root cause of it. Eventually, he flees into the waiting arms of the quacks, who 'hurry on the bad symptoms with double rapidity' by selling him a vast array of conflicting and noxious remedies. As he becomes more and more exhausted by both the anxiety and the results of all of these medications, the patient flits between doctor, quack and the occasional 'old lady' with her 'family nostrums'. Eventually, he will either 'sink into a fixed melancholy' or abandon all faith in medical practitioners and swallow no more remedies. In this latter course of action, Moore says with startling honesty, lies his best chance of recovery.

Even though the organs of the hypochondriac region are still considered to be at fault for all of this, there is something so recognisable about this description of a hypochondriac's attempts to cure what ails them. The frustration with the dismissal of symptoms as imaginary, the restless shifting between different doctors in hope of receiving different diagnoses, the appeal to 'quacks' to provide a solution where more official, recognised medicine has failed – this could be an account of me today and you tomorrow.

Moore is also refreshingly clear-eyed about the role that his own colleagues, the qualified doctors, play in the hypochondriac's progress. If a highly successful society doctor can expect to earn about £3,000 a year from his profession, he says, then a 'moderate computation' suggests that around £2,500 of that income will derive from 'prescribing for imaginary complaints, or such as would have disappeared fully as soon as they had been left to themselves'. In other words, hypochondriacs account for over eighty per cent of such a doctor's income. But the doctor is not to be blamed for this, he argues, nor is this something to be denigrated. If such visits and prescriptions provide comfort and reassurance to a patient, is that not also a form of care? I only wish Moore could have been present for the debate that was to come in the twentieth century around whether 'humouring' hypochondriacs like this did more harm than good.

Unlike some of the other medical writers of his century, Moore is phlegmatic about the impact that medicine can have on a patient population mired in uncertainty and quackery – perhaps his humours tended in the cold, wet direction, although to say so would have been hopelessly outdated by the time he was practising. Doing nothing, he argued, can in some cases of illness and injury be almost as good as doing something:

> The difference between a good physician and a bad one is certainly very great; but the difference between a good physician and no physician at all, in many cases, is very little.

This still rings true: I cannot count the times that I have been to see the doctor, only to be told that the best thing to do is nothing at all. This is hard advice to receive, as Moore's patient with his imaginary illnesses clearly also finds, since it sends him to seek alternative opinions. The human craving for satisfying narrative demands an explanation for our suffering; to find a connection between all our disparate and worrying symptoms requires action: *do something*, it screams. Make an appointment, swallow a pill, take a test, tell a friend. Anything to avoid sitting with this anxiety in the awkward stasis of not knowing. Doing nothing requires a level of trust in the inner processes of the human body and medicine's understanding of them that most of us do not have. Like an overly exacting teacher pointing out failures but never praising successes, we are inclined to remember only the times when our bodies have let us down. Why would I trust my body to heal itself unaided when, left to its own devices, it has previously developed tumours?

It is from this desire to take action that quacks, or those wishing to exploit the desperate, have always derived their power. As Moore suggests, when the conventional medicine of the day cannot satisfy – the doctors are sceptical of the hypochondriac's symptoms, perhaps, or they cannot pinpoint the cause, or their treatments have no impact – the patient looks elsewhere.

Where does quackery end and 'proper' medicine begin? It is very difficult to say, since as we have already seen, the empirical or scientific tradition emerged from and was overlapped by far less evidence-based convictions about the power of belief and spirituality to heal. Even as a more official and codified way of treating common complaints came into being, there were always those who dissented or harked back to a previous mode of thinking. Thus, the dissemination of dubious remedies was already an entrenched companion to medicine by the eighteenth century. Quacks were working street corners 2,000 years before in Ancient Rome, scooping up custom from those too poor or too sceptical to visit the official physicians or temple healers. Just as hypochondria has morphed and changed with the world, so too at every stage of medical advancement has there been an outsider offering a seductive-sounding alternative treatment, at a price.

But what is a quack, really? The precise origins of the word itself are hard to pin down, but it is thought that the contemporary definition of 'a person who dishonestly claims to have medical or surgical skill, or who advertises false or fake remedies' derives from the Dutch word *kwakzalver*, which originally denoted a seller of salves for cysts or, more generally, home remedies, 'who walks about the place advertising his own concocted medicines by shouting'. The subsequent

English term has been used fluidly since the 1500s: on some occasions, a quack is defined narrowly as a fraudulent medical practitioner or salesman who knowingly misleads or deceives customers as to the nature of their treatment, and at other times it is used generally to denote anyone advocating a remedy not accepted by conventional medicine, even in good faith.

Quackery participates in the history and tradition of medicine too, just as hypochondria does. A common trope of quackery is the supposed rediscovery of 'long lost' remedies from ages past, as if therapeutic ideas can grow in strength and flavour with the passage of years like a fine wine. In this murky world of cravings and uncertainties, the grass is always greener – the bizarre remedies of another age seeming more attractive than those of your own. Thus, the quacks of Imperial Rome liked to reference the medicine of the Greek doctors from prior centuries, like Hippocrates and Polybus, and their counterparts of Renaissance England were obsessed with Ancient Egypt, prescribing the Hippocrates-era remedy of a warm, dry diet and lifestyle for epilepsy to counteract the excess of cold, wet phlegm that they understood to cause the condition. And in our own time, you can book a luxury trip to Mexico to take part in a *temazcal* ceremony, a kind of group meditation inside a 'house of heat' or sweat lodge that was practised by Mesoamerican tribes for centuries and is now marketed at upscale travellers as a way to feel more 'empowered'.

Beyond just mimicking or appropriating the traditional practices of other cultures, there is even evidence that at one time hypochondriacs were instructed to directly imbibe the surviving artefacts of ages past as part of their quest for health. One John Hall, son-in-law to William Shakespeare and a practitioner of medicine who held no formal medical degree, even went so far as to include embalmed Egyptian remains as an ingredient in his remedies as a way of ensuring direct connection with the curative powers of the past. In his case notes, written in Latin in the first quarter of the seventeenth century, he records being summoned to the bedside of a William Fortesque, aged twenty, who was 'troubled with the Falling-sickness, by consent from the Stomach, as also Hypochondriack Melancholy, with a depravation of both Sense and Motion of the two middle Fingers of the Right-hand'. Hall prescribed, among other things, inhaling a vapour made by burning a mixture of benzoin, black pitch, juice of rue and powdered mummy. Noxious and sacrilegious as it may sound to us now, it was deemed effective: Fortesque recovered quickly and was still free from his hypochondriacal preoccupations and the paralysis in his hand ten years later. Whether this was because of the medicinal power of the cremated Egyptian artefact, or some other cause, remains unclear. Perhaps William Fortesque's belief in the millennia-old power of the mummy was the crucial factor.

The fact that 'quack' is the noise that ducks make is telling in this context: until the invention of the printing press, the only tool a quack had for marketing their wares was their voice, and so they were, as the name suggests, inherently noisy. A quack was a performer, putting on a show to convince curious bystanders and hypochondriacs alike of the health benefits to be found in their products. The showmanship was part of the allure, and it still is. Why pay a qualified physician to tell you to come back in a week if it still hurts when you could instead today swallow a tonic that fizzes on its way to the stomach or apply a cream that changes colour on the skin? The more dramatic the effect, the more we think it works; hence the lure of the staggering before and after photographs in dodgy advertisements and the addition of a strong chemical smell to products that have no need for it. The allure of this theatrical quality to medicine has long been debated; it is far from a new concern. In one of Plato's Socratic dialogues, the speakers are concerned with the potential harm a skilled practitioner of rhetoric could do if they used their power to perform to convince an unsuspecting person of their medical prowess. Gorgias, a so-called sophist, gives an example of just how persuasive they could be:

> If a rhetorician and a doctor were to enter any city you please, and there had to contend in speech before the Assembly or some other meeting as to which of the two should be appointed physician, you would find the physician was nowhere, while the master of speech would be appointed if he wished.

It is not entirely comfortable to admit how much irrelevant details like confidence, carriage and body language matter to our perception of a medical practitioner, or how much the taste or appearance of a remedy inclines us to believe in its effectiveness, but it is certainly the case. An accurate assessment of medical prowess is hard for a layperson to pull off, especially during a quick encounter. It is much easier to fuse our beliefs about clinical skill with that nebulous thing of a 'good bedside manner' and decide whether to trust a doctor because they stick the needle in confidently straight away, rather than stare at the injection site for a while to determine the best angle. A patient's demeanour and body language matter too: I am sure I am taken more seriously in medical examinations because of my accent, my whiteness and my middle-class confidence.

Even when the treatment on offer is entirely rooted in

scientific research, putting one's life in the hands of a stranger is still a matter of faith, and the patient must have some basis upon which to make this leap of faith. Given this, it's very easy to see how a charismatic fraudster with a compelling manner could be taken as a bona fide doctor without any question, either in Socratic-era Greece or in modern Britain. A case in point: I just took a sneaky break from writing this section to check the news, and was confronted with a startlingly ancient yet contemporary story about how a clinical psychiatrist who had practised in the UK for over two decades had been found to have forged her medical qualifications. Despite the letter of verification that came with her fake certificate misspelling the word 'verify', she was admitted to the official register of medical practitioners by the General Medical Council in the 1990s and worked unimpeded for the NHS for twenty years before she was caught in 2018 attempting to change an elderly patient's will in her favour. The quacks of centuries past would have been rather impressed by this, I think.

The impersonation of genuine medical practitioners or other authority figures has always been a major component of quackery, especially in the period when medicine was not yet well established or regulated. One amusing, or horrifying, example comes in the shape of Joshua Ward, a former pickle seller from the banks of the Thames, who made a name for himself in France in the early 1700s by selling a pair of remedies that he claimed could cure all human ailments. Upon his return to England he successfully masqueraded as the Member of Parliament for Marlborough for several months before being discovered and struck from the records of the House of Commons. He fell back on his medical wheeze, and quickly turned 'Ward's Pill and Drop' into a city-wide sensation, even though its main effect on a sick person was to make them much sicker. The pill was made from a compound of the toxic metalloid antimony, which would be fatal if taken in sufficient quantity, while the drop could only claim to effect a cure in the sense that it would immediately make the patient lose the entire contents of their stomach, perhaps taking other toxins with it. It would have undoubtedly felt like the medication was *doing something*, though, which perhaps explains its popularity. Despite the poisonous nature of his wares, Ward had many fans – including the novelist Henry Fielding – and the Royal Navy even stocked his Pill and Drop on their ships for nautical emergencies.

As Ward's example demonstrates, just being skilled at impersonation is not sufficient for a quack – they must also have a product onto which the hypochondriac tendencies of potential customers could project reassurance and safety. This is amply demonstrated by the lesson of one memorable medical swindler, a Mrs Joanna Stephens, who arrived in London in 1735 and quickly became a popular purveyor of a remedy for 'the stone'. Bladder and kidney stones were a common and painful complaint among the upper classes, whose meat-rich diet made them much more susceptible to these mineral deposits in the urinary system than those eating sparser, more plant-based peasant food. Without a drug that could reduce uric acid levels or safe surgery, the stone could easily prove fatal, which goes some way to explaining why Mrs Stephens' remedy was so sought after by the desperate. After repeated requests – and no doubt scenting an opportunity to bring off the scam of the century – she declared that if £5,000 (over half a million pounds today) was raised for her so that she could retire from business and move to the country, she would reveal the recipe. Over £1,300 came in from private individuals, and then, astonishingly, a committee of parliament was formed to find the rest from the public coffers, it being felt that having this remedy in the public domain was in the national interest.

Mrs Stephens kept her side of the bargain. Once she received her money, she arranged for the recipe to be published in *The Gentleman's Magazine*. It read:

> The Pills consist of Snails calcined, wild carrott seeds, burdock seeds, ashen keys, hips and hawes – all burnt to blackness – Alicant soap and honey.

Needless to say, Mrs Stephens disappeared with her money and was never heard of again. And the mystique that had had so many high-class clients swearing that her remedy for the stone worked brilliantly vanished with her. Once they knew that they were ingesting burnt snails mixed with soap and honey, her clients found that the remedy didn't seem to be so effective anymore. It was the mystery and the story that had made it feel like it was working, and without that it did nothing at all.

It is only relatively recently that there has been a robust (albeit imperfect) framework to ensure that doctors are qualified and medicinal drugs are regulated. In the US, the earliest attempts at regulation occurred in New York in the 1680s, when a colonial law prohibited practising 'without the advice and consent of such as are skillful in the said Arts'. After the US gained independence then passed the Tenth Amendment in 1791, the issue was devolved from a federal to a state level – a system that is still upheld today, with state medical boards across the country setting and upholding licence conditions for doctors. Things were very different in the UK, going back even a hundred years to the time of the First World War. There was no such thing as the NHS, doctors' services had to be paid for out of pocket, and concerned families could freely buy hampers at Harrods that contained heroin and cocaine to send to loved ones serving in the trenches. Go back another century, when there was not yet a General Medical Council to scrutinise doctors' qualifications or continued fitness to practise, and Britain was living through what one historian has described as 'an age of pills and potions', and the boundaries were even more blurred.

Even the Royal College of Physicians, which had been founded in 1518 to draw clear lines between medicine and quackery, was rather murky in its practices. Its original charter vowed that members would work 'to curb the audacity of those wicked men who shall profess medicine more for the sake of their avarice than from the assurance of any good conscience, whereby many inconveniences may ensue to the rude and credulous populace'. While some of these official, accredited physicians undoubtedly had noble intentions, their Royal Charter also gave the college the power to apprehend, put on trial and punish anyone found to be practising medicine or selling remedies outside of the college's authority – which was both a means of stemming the flood of suspicious remedies and a handy way of eliminating competition from apothecaries and community healers. This is what keeps that seed of doubt forever growing for the hypochondriac: doctors, even the properly trained ones, are human too, and subject to the same mistakes and vices as the rest of us. Medicine was a business, degree certificates could be bought and the interests of the college had to be safeguarded.

It is true that there were the unmistakable fraudsters, like Joanna Stephens and the Elizabethan astrologer and herbalist Simon Forman – consulted by Robert Burton – who claimed to have discovered that the ultimate cure for a woman's sexual dysfunction was a night between the sheets with him. But the medical regulators of the seventeenth and eighteenth centuries also looked askance at the likes of Sarah Mapp, a bonesetter of great renown who practised in the 1720s and 1730s. There seems to have been no question about Mapp's skill at her art. Her father had also been a bonesetter, and the combination of this education with her own physical strength – she was, for the time, an unusually large and strong woman – made her ideally suited to treating musculoskeletal injuries. She was so in demand that the town of Epsom in Surrey, where she lived, paid her an annual stipend of £100 to remain there, because the foot traffic her clinic attracted was so good for the local economy. Mapp did make the fifteen mile journey to London by coach twice a week, though, where she would establish herself for the day in the Grecian Coffee House by Wapping Old Stairs and wait for patients to come to her.

She had an acrimonious relationship with the physicians of the Royal College, whom she looked down on for their lack of practical knowledge of the human body. Humours, vapours and other fluids held no interest for her: everything she knew about treating people's problems she learned with her eyes and her hands. To her, the human body must have seemed like a purely mechanical entity, with parts that could become broken or misaligned. There was little need to study theory when she could fix someone with a well-placed wrench of a bone back into a socket. The theorists, in their turn, were scornful of Mapp's rough and ready approach to treatment, her lack of scholarship and her enormous popularity among the people most likely to injure themselves in this way – manual labourers. What she did was never going to be accepted as 'medicine' by the official authorities, yet hundreds of people benefited from it.

The conflict between Sarah Mapp and the college was emblematic of the larger struggle going on at this time between formal and informal medicine. For instance, Sarah fixed a spinal injury in a niece of Sir Hans Sloane, president of both the Royal Society and the Royal College of Physicians, impressing that gentleman and casting doubt on their previous characterisation of her as a mere quack. The doctors, eager to show her up some-how, sent her a patient who pretended to have a damaged wrist. Sarah, spotting the deception immediately, dislocated his per-fectly sound joint herself and told him to go back and 'have it set by the fools who had sent him'. Towards the end of her life, Sarah Mapp fell into alcoholism and an unfortunate marriage with an unscrupulous footman. She became known as 'Crazy Sally' and her reputation was further dented by her inclusion in William Hogarth's popular 1736 satirical engraving deploring quacks, which he titled 'The Company of Undertakers' in a pointed dig at the survival rate of their patients. She died the following year in poverty and obscurity, her bonesetter's art obscured by misogyny and accusations of quackery.

The chequered career of Sarah Mapp spoke to a dynamic in medicine that still exists. Medicine is a fallible, human institution, and as such is subject to the biases and prejudices of the people who have shaped it. It has always been the case that some practitioners that operate outside its structures have integrity and value, while others are knowingly or unknow-ingly peddling harmful and useless material. Some so-called quacks, who travelled constantly to find patients, put on their show and sell their wares, amassed a much broader experience and understanding of the human body than those with medi-cal degrees, who tended to serve those wealthy enough to pay them and prioritise the Hippocratic and Galenic versions with little reference to empirical study. Paracelsus, the Swiss physi-cian and philosopher credited with introducing observation as a powerful tool of early modern science, spent years travelling around Europe to gather this kind of knowledge before taking a position at a university. 'A doctor must seek out old wives, gypsies, sorcerers, wandering tribes, old robbers, and such outlaws and take lessons from them. A doctor must be a traveller ... Knowledge is experience,' he wrote later. And many discerning patients preferred the treatment of this less academic kind of doctor. The philosopher Thomas Hobbes once said 'I would rather have the advice, or take physick from an experienced old woman that had been at many sick people's bedsides than from the learnedst but inexperienced physician.'

It has certainly been my experience that some of the most comforting and compassionate treatment I have received has come not from those with the most eminent medical qualifications. In the meeting where I was told I had cancer, it was the nurse, not the doctor, who sprang forward to catch my mother as she fainted and took her away to lie down. There is a healing power in a kind, experienced touch that cannot be surpassed. I still remember what it felt like when, during a horrible gynaecological procedure at a teaching hospital that was being witnessed by half a dozen male medical students, the nurse assisting held on to my ankle for the whole thing, squeezing in sympathy every time the doctor prolonged the ordeal so he could demonstrate another technique.

Some of what quacks had to offer was dung mixed with honey and sold in a fancy bottle, and some of it was based in the properties of plants upon which modern pharmacology still draws today. Some of it worked and some of it didn't. The same could be said of the official physicians' prescriptions too. One Dr Dover, a pupil of Thomas Sydenham, became known as 'Dr Quicksilver' in the early 1700s because he believed that mercury – which is toxic to all systems of the body even upon brief exposure – could cure all ills and prescribed it to his patients constantly. He was no quack, according to the working definition of that word at the time. He possessed a bona fide medical degree and would easily have passed muster at a Royal College of Physicians inspection. No wonder confusion reigned. What can a concerned hypochondriac do, other than keep trying it all? The doubt and the hope forever dwell in the possibility that this pill, this tincture, this cordial, will be the one that makes the difference. And, just like Hobbes, we are still inclined to trust experience over theory. I can think of countless times when a recommendation from a friend or a particularly emphatic online review has finally convinced me to try something that my doctor has been recommending for months, or has pushed me into purchasing a supplement with little or no evidential backing for its claims. I would classify my years-long obsession with iron in my early twenties under this heading; I have never been anaemic, although I came close during some of my cancer treatment, yet after a colleague at my first journalism job was diagnosed with severe iron deficiency I became fixated on the idea that I must have it too. The constant presence on the London Underground of an advert for an iron supplement that featured a yawning woman and the slogan 'Tired of being tired?' didn't help me to talk myself out of this, either. I spent a lot of time researching and then purchasing remedies claiming to boost iron levels without any hard evidence either that they worked or that I needed them. This impulse goes beyond the rational. It is wholly hypochondriacal.

Accompanying all of this compulsive consumption of quackery was the powerful force that is fashion. When I think of the eighteenth century, my imagination immediately conjures up a time peopled by bewigged aristocrats in satin breeches snorting and guzzling the latest remedy for whatever ailed them, partly because they believed it would make them feel better and partly because it was in vogue. At this point, the taste in quackery tended towards cure-alls – panaceas that, it was claimed, could treat all manner of different conditions with just the one medication. It's an incredibly seductive idea, and one that I still encounter regularly today in the form of probiotic supplements or herbal remedies like echinacea and cannabidiol (CBD) that claim to boost the immune system and effect all kinds of holistic wonders from a single substance. Just take this one little pill and everything that ails you will be vanquished. Fairy tales and folklore are full of this moment: a potion to be swallowed that will transform or destroy a life. I think of Alice picking up the bottle labelled 'drink me' and wondering if it is poison, before draining it to the dregs anyway. When life is especially complicated or hard, the notion that just a single action could render everything straightforward and easy is especially attractive. This is part of our wider impulse to narrativise. The hardships must mean something. The cure must be dramatic and all-encompassing, because incremental or intermittent improvement makes for a terrible story. Alice did not shrink gradually.

These panaceas had names that spoke to their dramatic potential to transform a previously miserable existence: Turlington's Balsam of Life, Wessel's Jesuit's Drops, Bromfield's Pilulae in Omnes Morbos and Lucas's Pure Drops of Life were just a few of the many hundreds of such remedies on offer. Chief among them was the soothingly named 'Cordial Balm of Gilead', a treatment for a barely defined malady sold by a medical pretender and entrepreneur named Samuel Solomon. The fascinating thing about Solomon was how seamlessly he had transitioned the tenets of traditional quackery into the age of the printing press and the pamphlet while seeming to hold himself aloof from the rough and tumble of the cure-all market. He spent thousands of pounds on advertising in newspapers and periodicals, but not for his product directly. Instead, he presented himself as a philosopher and sought readers for his *A Guide to Health*, a meandering text that borrowed very heavily from Robert Burton's *The Anatomy of Melancholy*. Only once the reader was fully immersed in it would they realise that all of Solomon's philosophical questions pointed towards just one answer: the Cordial Balm of Gilead, which the author conveniently offered for sale by the bottle via a mail order service. At no point in the *Guide* is there a clear description of the condition that the Balm treats, though. It can be used against 'nervous disorders, juvenile indiscretions, head-aches, debility, seminal weakness, lowness of spirits, female complaints, loss of appetite, relaxation, indigestion, coughs and colds, consumptions, weaknesses, impurity of blood', among other things.

Solomon himself tried to embody all kinds of medical practitioner in one. He would proudly boast, in the tradition of Paracelsus, that practical experience trumped theory and that many important medical advances had been made by those outside the narrow confines of officialdom – a lethal blend of fiction and fact. At the same time, he masqueraded as a qualified doctor, claiming to have 'regularly graduated' from a university and presenting himself in his advertisements as the holder of an MD. He was the ultimate quack, borrowing and combining different kinds of authority to convince the anxious that he held all the answers. And he was not above harnessing the power of hypochondria directly to drum up more custom, either. 'Nervous and hypochondriacal complaints resist ... all remedies ... except the famous and highly-exalted medicine, the Cordial Balm of Gilead,' he declared. This feels like Solomon's master stroke to me, simultaneously acknowledging that hypochondria is a major reason why someone might be exploring alternatives to conventional medicine while also insisting that only his product can provide relief. The lure of this kind of confident authority and certainty is intense, especially for someone who feels shunned or ridiculed by their official medical providers, and it made Solomon very wealthy. A large bottle of the Cordial Balm of Gilead cost a guinea – a week's wages for a skilled tradesman at the time and equivalent to around £50 today – and it was, coincidentally, recommended that it be taken at least three times a day. Forever chasing the latest panaceas for hypochondria was a very expensive business, and it still is. Reassurance, even the temporary kind offered by the likes of Solomon, always comes at a price.

Quackery has changed since its heyday in the eighteenth century. Rather than defining itself against science, in the nineteenth century it began to adopt the same language and ideas. Laypeople were now more aware of the scientific method and advancements in evidence-based medicine, and thus far less likely to believe that one tonic could cure both a headache and gout as well as everything in between. Panaceas were out and specifics were in. By the middle of the century, remedies were far more likely to target particular complaints, so that someone might take one set of pills for their stomach problems, another for their skin rashes and yet another for their feelings of anxiety. Treatments for aesthetic issues like baldness, weight and height also became a major tenet of quackery as ideas of health fused with certain beauty standards and ideals.

This was the origin of what we today call 'wellness', a multi-trillion-dollar industry that thrives on the same aspects of hypochondria as the quackery of old. Looking back to the frontispiece to Robert Burton's *The Anatomy of Melancholy*, we see everything we need to know about this shiny, modern, startup-ridden, disrupter-friendly capitalist playground. Now, an aura of medical authority, rather than mystical power, is what we crave in our quackery. Pills come in uncluttered, minimalist packaging that boasts of endorsements by experts and references to studies that show how this particular regimen has been linked to the adoption of healthier habits. One of my most avid fixations of the past few years has been the scandal surrounding the medical technology company Theranos, which was founded in 2003 by the nineteen-year-old college dropout Elizabeth Holmes, who claimed to have found a way to miniaturise and automate blood tests, so that results could be derived very quickly from tiny samples. By 2013, the company was valued at $10 billion and Holmes was acclaimed as a groundbreaking female entrepreneur. As was later exposed by researchers and journalists, there was never any evidence that Theranos could deliver on its promise of near-instant diagnosis for a whole host of conditions, but so powerfully attractive was its offering of a revolutionary medical advance with greater certainty about health that the company operated for over a decade before the truth came to wider attention. Theranos finally shut down in 2018 and its founder was found guilty of fraud in 2022. It is the most potent example of our age, I think, of just how powerful the hypochondriac impulse can be. The desire to be able to know what ails us immediately, with just a finger prick of blood, was so strong that an entire industry overlooked the deep flaws in the science behind this supposed advancement. The most telling detail of all is that Holmes' original name for the company was 'Real-Time Cures'. There is nothing a hypochondriac wants more.

Part of what makes Theranos a timeless morality tale for this condition is the sheer volume of money it made. There has always been a strong link between the hypochondriac and the contents of their purse. Among the engravings that show different embodiments of melancholy in Burton's book, 'Hypochondriacus' – clearly a rich man of elevated social status – reclines dejectedly in a fur-lined robe. His head rests on his hand as he contemplates the profusion of medicine bottles and unravelling recipe scrolls around him, none of which seem to have alleviated what ails him. The image cleverly conveys two things that are fundamental to the contemporary understanding of the hypochondriac: they want treatment and they are willing to spend money on it, as the fancy robe and the no doubt expensive array of remedies demonstrate.

The fact that Hypochondriacus looks so good – his hat is flattering, his beard is well groomed – even while he feels terrible is important. Ideas of sickness and health have always been connected with appearance. Even from the earliest days of the human evolutionary journey, we have been programmed to visually detect subtle signs of ill health in others and keep our distance. But at certain times in history, changing conceptions of beauty – and mostly it is female beauty – have complicated our ability to judge what is healthy.

From the late eighteenth century onwards, the ideal of female attractiveness came to be overlaid with tuberculosis-inspired aesthetics of sickness: the pallor, the slender frame, the heightened colour in the cheeks. Gone was the interest of previous eras in a generous, well-nourished female form; now the most attractive a woman could be was to look as if she was literally wasting away. Ann Radcliffe's 1791 Gothic novel *The Romance of the Forest* was an early trendsetter in this arena, seamlessly merging sexuality and fragility in its description of Adeline, a damsel in distress who has fainted just a few lines earlier:

Her beauty, touched with the languid delicacy of illness, gained from sentiment what it lost in bloom. The negligence of her dress, loosened for the purpose of freer respiration, discovered those glowing charms, which her auburn tresses, that fell in profusion over her bosom, shaded, but could not conceal.

By the second half of the nineteenth century, a 'cult of invalidism' had taken root, especially among middle-class women, who viewed the creative potential of their illnesses as an escape from the restrictions of real life. The link between this fashionable frailty and devastating disease was strong and troubling. In January 1849, in a letter to her literary editor, Charlotte Brontë wrote from the side of her sister Anne's sickbed that 'consumption, I am aware, is a flattering malady'. Four months later, Anne was dead of tuberculosis.

When I first started to be allowed to choose my own clothes as a pre-teen at the very end of the 1990s, all of the fashion I encountered was inspired by similar ideas to this. The 'heroin chic' of earlier in the decade, which prioritised pale skin, visible ribs, an emaciated frame and sunken eyes, had trickled down into the bargain retailers in which I was browsing. Low-slung trousers that exposed the hip bones and velvet ribbon chokers were everywhere. Showing off the delicacy of one's bones seemed like the only way to fit in, only where some girls had concave stomachs and androgynous figures, I possessed a chubby roundness that would have fared better in a less consumptive era of clothing.

The books I read at this time did not help to give me a more balanced view of things. I was – and still am – a huge fan of the Chalet School books by Elinor M. Brent-Dyer, a series of fifty-eight books that were published between 1925 and 1970. The first dozen or so were what caused me to fall in love: focused on an English boarding school situated by a beautiful lake in the Austrian Tyrol, they detailed the adventures of its pupils as they learned German, climbed mountains and performed plays. In many ways, they are typical of the school stories of the interwar period as produced by writers like Angela Brazil and Elsie J. Oxenham. But alongside all the usual jolly hockey sticks antics standard in this genre, the Chalet School books had something else too. They placed a great emphasis on health, and in later books the school was even connected to a tuberculosis sanatorium, with many of the pupils having parents or siblings undergoing treatment there. One of the central characters, the younger sister of the headmistress, is described from the outset as 'delicate', and a regular subplot involves her getting slightly wet on a rainy walk and then almost dying from a fever. Much is made in all of the books of categorising girls into those who are sturdy and sound in contrast to those who are of a flimsier constitution. These latter girls are constantly told that they must not overtire themselves and endanger their health. Plenty of fresh air, rich milk, cold baths and afternoon naps are prescribed at all times – standard aspects of the 'rest cure' of the early twentieth century. The books also dwelt lovingly on the forbearance and beauty of those girls who were never strong enough to fully take part in real life. They wore attractive bed jackets, bore their misfortunes with patient grace and were beloved by their families. In other words, the books fetishised the idea of the perfect invalid, and somehow this stuck fast in my brain. Even today, when I'm feeling especially burnt out or run down, I think fondly of the lifestyle these books espoused and wonder what it would take for me, too, to be rosy-cheeked and sturdy like the characters who always save the day in the nick of time.

*

'You look well,' a friend will say as you arrive at the restaurant and remove your coat. What is it that prompts this remark? A certain confidence of posture, perhaps, or a glow to the skin. Something superficial or different, like a new haircut or a well-fitting shirt in a flattering colour. Most of the time, this is greeted as the casual compliment that the speaker intends, and the world continues to turn. Thanks, I've been sleeping well recently, I might reply. What shall we order? But when you are not well, or believe that you are not well, this exchange becomes fraught with meaning, most of it uncomfortable. For me, there are three scenes that play in my mind when I think about this, unbidden, like a roll of film unspooling across the floor.

Scene one. I'm in my last year of school and, unbeknown to me, I already have cancer. I'm putting books back on a high shelf in a classroom, reaching up so that my jacket lifts and exposes my waist. I hear a voice behind me: it's one of the sporty, thin, shiny-haired girls whom I have spent six years sharing classes with yet never spoken to. She is inviting me to walk to lunch with her and complimenting me on how well my diet is working. I feel instantly queasy – I'm not dieting, intentionally, but food often makes me feel like I'm going to vomit and all my clothes are now loose – but I push the feeling down in favour of the excitement of being singled out by someone popular. Similar invitations come in the days and weeks that follow. Would I like to skive lessons and drive to McDonald's to share one tiny packet of French fries with three other girls instead? Can I come to town to give my opinion on a range of, to me, entirely interchangeable clothing options for an upcoming party? Will I sit with the popular girls on the bus? Suddenly, I am accelerating up the school's social hierarchy in a baffling manner, all because I am mysteriously becoming thinner. Once that mystery is solved, though, and the news of my cancer leaks out, my stock plummets again. This rapid rise and fall through the very clearly delineated social structures of my all-girls school adds a dizzying dimension to the whole ordeal, and it takes me years to unpack what has really happened.

Scene two. A few months after my diagnosis, I'm standing in the deputy headteacher's office, helping her look through a filing cabinet for some paperwork I need in order to apply for a medical exemption to some exams I will be unable to take because I'm now undergoing cancer treatment. Steroids have made my face puffy and there is an itchy wig pulled down hard over my bald head. I think it looks like black straw, obviously fake in colour, texture and shape, but in a vain attempt to improve matters this morning I tied a wide blue ribbon around it as a kind of headband. Mrs Williams finds a promising document, a letter from my doctor outlining the likely progress of my condition and treatment, and starts quickly reading aloud the list of symptoms to me to confirm that she has the right piece of paper for my application. 'Nausea, fatigue, muscle loss, hair loss …' she murmurs, her glance flicking over me. 'Well, you've been lucky there, your hair looks the same as ever,' she says. The wig prickles at the nape of my neck and I flush. I blurt out that I am wearing a wig made of plastic, and the silence that follows is very awkward. I thought the wig automatically showed everybody that I had cancer, but here is someone who has known me since I was eleven years old saying that it looks just like my real hair did back when I was healthy. I don't know what to think.

Scene three. I'm in the hallway at my parents' house, watching one of my best friends walk through the front door. It's been a year since I left school for university and I have just been discharged from my longest hospital stay to date – three weeks in an isolation room in London so that I could receive a stem cell transplant. My immune system has been judged to have recovered sufficiently to allow visitors. 'You look great,' she says, hugging my once-more angular body tightly. 'Being this size suits you.' I know she is being nice, but I think of the sixteen days in the last month that I spent unable to eat anything but a single teaspoon of yoghurt, and how the chemotherapy destroyed the lining of my mouth and throat so that anything I put in it burns. By the time she lets go of me, my smile has become stiff and fake.

I still don't know what my adult body looks like when it is healthy. Thanks to a constantly shifting combination of treatments, illnesses and lifestyle changes since I was seventeen, I have been a whole variety of sizes. I own clothes that fit inside each other like Russian dolls. I had thick, light-brown straight hair, then I had thinner, almost black curly hair, and now I have some unremarkable combination of the two.

The aesthetics of modern wellness fascinate me: the pastel corporate branding, the emphasis on 'clean' eating; the 'Pilates body'; superfoods; raw, plant-based ingredients; and 'activated' elements. It is the Hippocratic regimen of centuries past repackaged for a new age, the panacea given a new form. Everything changes, and nothing changes.

The emphasis on the clean and the natural, in food, skincare, make-up and more, is especially enthralling for the hypochondria-inclined consumer. Attaining the truly high level of health that many of us feel must be locked away inside us somewhere, obscured by toxins and germs, is a tantalising goal. And this is what so many of the companies and influencers who operate in this $4.4 trillion global industry purport to offer: a chance to unlock the 'real' you, who is truly *well*. Everything, from Gwyneth Paltrow's zany Goop brand to the customised vitamin subscriptions that sponsor half the podcasts I listen to, is aimed at selling this vision.

So much of it is gendered too. Social media is swimming with images of lean, toned women posing in athletic clothing and extolling the benefits of gratitude journalling every morning at sunrise and wearing expensive make-up that makes it look like you just have bare skin that glows with visible health. This is overwhelmingly aimed at women; women who must spend money and mental effort to alter every aspect of their lives so as to align with the wellness goals that they have imbibed. Everything becomes commodified in this world. Even something as basic and necessary as drinking water becomes surrounded by potential purchases: what kind of bottle we are drinking from, what drops or powders we are adding, what devices we are using to keep it at the perfect temperature. Of course, it is easy to find parallels between the appeal of this world and the quackery of previous eras. The motivation to *just do something* is strongly present in both, as is the lure of the dramatic transformation. But what marks out this current incarnation of these very old ideas is the shift in authority. Those peddling powders and pills are no longer assuming any kind of medical authority to lend prestige or mystique to their assertions. Instead, they spin the yarn that they are laypeople just like us, only slightly better because they have been using this treatment for a while now. How could you resist?

Why did the burnt snail concoction work for so many of the people who took Mrs Stephens' cure? For the same reason that it stopped working once the recipe was published and its bogus nature exposed: the powerful belief that what they were swallowing was effective medicine that would lessen their pain. This interaction of imagination and sensation had been identified by Michel de Montaigne back in 1572, in an essay in which he identified his own impressionability when it came to illness: 'As I observe a disease, so I catch it and give it lodging in myself,' he wrote. This same effect worked with treatment too, he went on to explain:

> Why do doctors begin by practising on the credulity of their patients with so many false promises of a cure, if not to call the powers of the imagination to the aid of their fraudulent concoctions? They know, as one of the masters of their craft has given it to them in writing, that there are men on whom the mere sight of medicine is operative.

The first attempt at a clinical trial of this effect was carried out in 1799 by a Dr John Haygarth of Bath, who was irked by the popularity of a quack medical device for pain and inflammation known as the 'Perkins tractor'. They had been created by a Dr Elisha Perkins of Connecticut – a bona fide doctor who had served as an army surgeon during the American War of Independence – and took the form of a small pointed metal rod that when waved over the affected body part, Perkins claimed, could 'draw off the noxious electrical fluid that lay at the root of suffering'. The exact makeup of these rods was a closely guarded secret, and the mystery of these devices coupled with the fact that Perkins claimed to have effected over 5,000 cures created a huge demand for the treatment in the US. Consequently, Perkins' son had brought the tractors to London and started selling them for five guineas each, quickly attracting customers from the very highest echelons of society.

The fact that the tractors had gained such an enthusiastic following 'even amongst persons of rank and understanding' prompted Haygarth to investigate. His motives were partly scientific curiosity and partly, no doubt, a combination of snobbishness and self-preservation. If the wealthy elite of Bath – a fashionable spa town with a booming medical trade – were preferring the Perkins tractor to the ministrations of ordinary physicians, this could prove to be a problem. Thus, Haygarth and a colleague at Bath General Hospital devised a trial of the tractors. They created two dummy devices out of wood, which looked identical to the real thing, and used them to 'treat' five patients with chronic rheumatism. The following day, they used the actual Perkins tractors in exactly the same way on the same people, and then compared their results. Four of the five found that their symptoms were relieved by the false devices, and there was no difference in outcome between the two days of tests. Haygarth published a pamphlet sharing the news that pieces of wood were just as effective as the expensive Perkins tractor. He even opined that doctors should harness the power of what he called 'medical faith' to bring relief to their patients – an idea that is only now gaining currency in medical research circles after many decades of trying to eliminate this imaginative variable from scientific study entirely.

The word 'placebo' already existed at the time that Haygarth was waving sticks over people's swollen knees, but it meant to please or flatter, drawn from the Latin word *placere*, to please. It wasn't applied to this effect until over 120 years later, when T. C. Graves published a paper in *The Lancet* in 1920 discussing the therapeutic effect or 'placebo effect' of a treatment that had previously been regarded sceptically. It became a common feature of medical research after the Second World War, when the American pharmacologist and anaesthetist Henry K. Beecher observed that the psychological status of returning service personnel seemed to influence their perception of pain.

Double-blind methods became common in drug trials, that is, the inclusion of a control group who receive a placebo without the knowledge of either the participants or the researchers, since more investigation showed that the words spoken or even the body language deployed by a physician can alert a patient to the fact that they are not receiving the drug. Performing better than a placebo became the gold standard for new drugs.

The placebo effect is most visible with conditions where perception and imagination are key to the experience, such as pain, fatigue, headache, anxiety and depression. To put it crudely, a sugar pill can't heal a broken leg, but it can affect your perception of how much it hurts. Montaigne had it right: if imagination can give you the sensation of a disease, then it can also give you a cure. And hypochondriacs, it would seem, are definitely susceptible to the placebo effect. In a double-masked placebo-controlled study of whether the antidepressant fluoxetine can be used to treat hypochondria, around thirty per cent of the participants receiving the placebo reported an improvement in their condition. The actual drug was even better – twice as effective, in fact – but one in three of those receiving no active ingredients at all also reported a positive outcome. This conforms with placebo rates across different types of trials, which generally stand between twenty and forty per cent. Those who imagine their illnesses are at least as likely as the general population to imagine their cure, then, which explains why there is such a long connection between hypochondria and obviously ineffective remedies.

Making use of the placebo effect poses an ethical dilemma. Its therapeutic value is well established, and it seems to be able to help in situations when there are few other available treatments – hypochondria, per the above study, being a good example of this. But lying to patients is not what doctors are meant to do, even if it is done with the best of intentions. There is evidence that this prohibition on deception is avoided by some physicians by prescribing what are called 'semi-placebos' such as vitamins or unnecessary antibiotics – a harmless dose of something that nevertheless gives the patient the sense that their condition is being treated and increases the chance of a positive reaction. Just in the last few years, though, so-called open-label placebos have been generating very interesting results. These are placebos administered 'without deception', with the patient fully informed that what they are taking contains no active ingredients or drugs of any kind. A 2020 study found that they had 'genuine psychobiological effects' when used to decrease emotional distress, measured through both patient self-reporting and a neural biomarker. There is even now a direct-to-consumer wellness product called 'Zeebo' that sells 'honest placebo pills' in which 'you are the active ingredient'. For $25, the customer receives forty-five branded cellulose pills and access to a tracking app where they can document any change in their symptoms. The pills are entirely unspecific, so they can be taken for any perceived sickness the patient prefers. Best practice for using them involves focusing on the symptom you want to treat, setting out your expectations for the treatment, designing your own regimen and frequency for the pills, and then following it.

There is something compelling yet baffling about this idea. As one reviewer on their website wrote: 'Zeebo is kind of weird, but in a mysterious way, empowering.' This might be the perfect medication for the hypochondriac. The showmanship and illusion that dominated the quackery of centuries past are stripped away, leaving just a plain white bottle that makes it absolutely clear it contains nothing of value at all. Except we are being asked to pay for it. Is this a scam? Perhaps. But, a contrarian voice in my head whispers, are a lot of the ways we try to alleviate our aches and pains not similarly empty of active ingredients, albeit not so blatant about it? The only thing Zeebo promises is to help you 'tap into the power of your mind and body' via the placebo effect. Should I pay for this? Probably not. Although maybe, under capitalism, the only way to activate a sense of value in one's own health is to part with cash.

6

All in My Head

It took a long time for me to even entertain the idea that I might be a hypochondriac. It is much easier to see in hindsight than it was in the moment. For so long, the monitoring I did of my health was subsumed by the routines of cancer treatment. But gradually, as I was released from further check-ups and I slowly grew more comfortable sharing mundane details about colds and sprains with loved ones, I came to realise that my level of interest in my fluctuating state of wellness was far from the norm. The sheer variety of procedures I had undergone in my late teens – from multiple instances of general anaesthesia to a stem cell extraction that saw my entire volume of blood pumped several times through a giant centrifuge – had given me a level of comfort with the rarer elements of medicine that was unusual. More than that, though, the awareness crept up on me that I spent so much more time and effort on this aspect of life than anyone else I knew, even though I supposedly had no active conditions requiring treatment. Meeting my husband was also a crucial turning point during this time; never before had I encountered someone so blissfully uninterested in blood tests and minor twinges. At some point, then, my responsible cancer survivor behaviour had morphed into something else. Rather than worrying about actual developments with my illness, the worry itself had become the problem.

When I first started seeking help for my health anxiety, I was told over and over again to write everything down. Part of this is an attempt to create a practical bulwark around my spiralling yet ephemeral fears: by keeping a record of every medical appointment I attend I create a diary of each doctor's visit to refer back to when my brain is twisting and distorting the memories of what I had been told about my body's latest mysteries. Together, these scribblings form a dossier of evidence that I can use against myself when the anxiety about illness is getting worse. Paging back through it, I can see that far from consuming my every waking thought, as it feels in the worst moments, I didn't actually have any of these episodes yesterday, or the day before, and the one this morning was just a faint twinge about a numb toe that passed quickly.

This practice also has a more intangible purpose. Keeping a written record of the thoughts that escalate into anxious episodes is a way of noting them without allowing them to overpower, of acknowledging their presence while keeping them at a safer distance. It also satisfies the hypochondriac's demand to be known, for the narrative to hang together at last and so be acknowledged as real. The contradictions of this tug at me all the time: this is the most secret and private part of myself, and yet it only begins to make sense when I pour it onto the page where others can read it. I never want to start writing, but once I've stabbed a few bad-tempered words onto the page I always begin to feel better. There's an itchy yet satisfying pain to doing it well that feels a lot like picking at a scab. Trying to describe a hypochondriacal episode accurately is very like the excavating, scooping-out sensation of attempting to tell a doctor what is wrong with me, except without the pressure that comes with knowing that my chances of validation and treatment rest on my every choice of word.

There is a growing recognition within medicine itself that the way sickness is written about can play a role in its treatment. Dr Rita Charon at Columbia University, who is a doctor of both medicine and literature, proposed in 2000 a concept called 'narrative medicine', which uses writing, reading and the tools of literary analysis to connect the isolated incidences of a patient's illness together into a story that helps their physician provide better treatment. Writing is a fundamental part of her ideas for improving the doctor–patient relationship. Both sides of that divide keep a written record of their perceptions of the process, which they share and discuss along the way. This helps a patient to feel heard and a doctor to 'bear witness' to their suffering beyond just being the source of answers to technical questions.

'A scientifically competent medicine alone cannot help a patient grapple with the loss of health or find meaning in suffering,' Charon wrote in a seminal 2001 journal article that unpacked her ideas. 'Along with scientific ability, physicians need the ability to listen to the narratives of the patient, grasp and honor their meanings, and be moved to act on the patient's behalf.' Doctors need what she terms 'narrative competence' as well as clinical prowess – 'that is, the competence that human beings use to absorb, interpret, and respond to stories'. The kind of listening that a doctor ought to be doing in a diagnostic setting is equivalent to reading a piece of literature with an open mind, she argues, and letting one's memories, imagination and interpretative powers assist in discovering meaning. Only then can good answers be found to a patient's fundamental questions about the narrative of the diagnosis they have received, like 'What is wrong with me' and 'What will become of me?' It sounds wonderful in theory, but I do have my doubts about how this might work in the everyday reality of a busy clinic: will any doctor have the time to do all of the listening, writing and thinking that this involves?

That moment in the consulting room when a patient first has to tell the story of their symptoms so that the doctor can write their history recalls the first time a reader opens a book and makes a connection with an author. This 'telling of the self', as Charon terms it, splits the patient in two: they are both the protagonist of the story as well as its author, creating a division similar to that experienced by the writer of an autobiography or memoir. I find this multiplication difficult enough to handle in the division between my professional self, a writer of memoir, and the rest of me – sometimes on the way to an event I rack my brain to remember which version of me has been invited. Sometimes my existence can feel like a film shot from multiple angles at once, all played together. There is the me who is sitting at her desk typing this now, then the version I am putting together on the page, and perhaps a nebulous third figure who is created in collaboration between me writing this and you reading it. The same is true in the consulting room. No wonder it feels like the body and the mind have separate agendas in this fragmented, disassociated state.

Finding the right language to shape our sensations is hard too, and without the words to describe them, it could be argued, our symptoms have yet to come into being. Do I hurt until I have told somebody else about the pain? Virginia Woolf lamented the dearth of reliable expressions for sickness in her 1926 essay 'On Being Ill'. Describing a patient's difficulty in conveying to his doctor the details of the condition that requires diagnosis, she resorts to visceral imagery that recalls illness itself. 'There is nothing ready made for him. He is forced to coin words himself, and, taking his pain in one hand, and a lump of pure sound in the other ... so to crush them together that a brand new word in the end drops out,' she wrote. This paucity of expression, Woolf argues, is responsible for a disappointing lack of literature about illness. 'English, which can express the thoughts of Hamlet and the tragedy of Lear, has no words for the shiver and the headache,' she says. She wrote the first version of this essay not long after experiencing a nervous breakdown that kept her in bed for weeks; her irritation that so much of the canon is devoted to love and romance rather than this, to her, more pressing experience, is palpable. 'Of all this daily drama of the body there is no record. People write always about the doings of the mind; the thoughts that come to it; its noble plans; how it has civilised the universe.' She is jealous of 'the merest schoolgirl', who, when looking to literature to help her express the overwhelming feelings of first love, 'has Shakespeare, Donne and Keats to speak her mind for her', whereas 'let a sufferer try to describe a pain in his head to a doctor and language at once runs dry'. These literary greats, she implies, neglected to put their linguistic powers in service of articulating illness, and the world is the poorer for it.

I disagree with Woolf. All three of the writers she names wrote brilliantly about illness, both their own and other people's, and in fact I find literature in general to be overflowing with accounts of sickness. The problem that I think she had, and that I have too, is not so much of word selection but of narrative veracity. It is impossible to condense every sensation and symptom into a believable account that someone else can understand. Feelings change second to second; I might wake up feeling better, then get worse a few hours later, then cheerfully get up for lunch before relapsing seriously mid-afternoon. How can all of this ever be condensed into a few words for the consumption of someone who has not experienced it, or anything like it? Talking about it, all the time, narrating in real time, is exhausting and can make you feel like a burden to loved ones and carers. When the doctor calls in the evening, I will curate the story of the day, picking the elements that I feel are most relevant. It is my illness, after all, and my story to tell. I have to make meaning of it. How well I do it, though, will determine how he perceives me and how he treats me. My status as a white, middle-class woman with a higher education will always ensure that I get a better hearing than someone without those advantages, especially when it comes to shaping the story of my symptoms into something plausible. Hypochondria is a perpetual act of this choosing, of living at all times in the act of deciding what version of yourself is least likely to attract ridicule or scorn.

A common accusation levelled at those who experience hypochondria is that we secretly enjoy the status and process of being ill. That consciously or unconsciously we desire the attention and focus it brings, and that symptoms appear only in order to prolong the sensation of being important. I worry, too, that others will see me as self-indulgent for allowing my thoughts about my health to dominate me, even though when I am experiencing such an episode it does not feel as if there is any choice to be made. I am not alone in this either. Self-described hypochondriac Immanuel Kant dwelt on this in *The Conflict of the Faculties*, arguing that reason and discipline are the antithesis of giving in to hypochondria:

The exact opposite of the mind's power to master its pathological feelings is hypochondria, the weakness of

abandoning oneself despondently to general morbid feelings
that have no definite object (and so making no attempt to
master them by reason).

For Kant, reason rules the hierarchy of our cognitive faculties, and the only way to eradicate hypochondria is to train
the mind in order that the weakness of the will that entertains
hypochondriacal thoughts is driven out. The mind is superior
to the body and, with sufficient effort, can govern how the two
interact. He kept himself on a strict regimen, inspired by Stoic
principles, that saw him 'alternate the mechanical occupation of
the stomach or the feet with the mental occupation of thinking'.
In this way, Kant seems to have kept his anxieties in check – he
was so precisely regular in his habits that his neighbours could
set their clocks by his daily cycle of walks. Perhaps he was
right, and those of us who have not succeeded in using reason
to govern our weaker impulses are merely lesser beings, lacking
the willpower to allow the mind to rule the body. Or perhaps
there is more to this than merely the ability to exert the will.

One person just as devoted as Kant to routine and daily ritual
was Charles Darwin, whose daily stroll along the sandwalk
behind his house in East Sussex (his 'thinking path' as he called
it) is now part of the mythology of how he came to write his
era-defining book about evolution, *On the Origin of Species*. But
there is a question over whether his rigid adherence to routine
was keeping his anxieties at bay or making them more acute.

I had already written about Charles Darwin's hypochondria,
I realised, long before I even knew the word for it. My very first
piece of published writing, at the age of twelve, was a poem
that won a competition in a youth arts magazine. It had been
inspired by a school trip to Darwin's residence, Down House,
where I had been shown the study in which he had thought and

read and written for hours every day. One corner was separated from the main room by a wooden screen, and the guide delicately mentioned that the bath, sink and privy that stood there were for his use during the work day, so he could 'sort himself out' without having to lose any time that should be spent in crafting *On the Origin of Species.*

The exact nature of Darwin's health problems was left vague, so I left that room with no more than a general sense that he liked to take a bath in the middle of the day, but everywhere else in the house was evidence of a man regulating his life against the paralysing fear of the unknown. There was the walk around the garden that he had timed precisely; the highly ordered daily timetable of work, meals and exercise; and the enormous grandfather clock that stood in the centre of the house, constantly filling it with the sound of time measured and time passing. I sat in this hallway, listening to the pendulum swinging, thinking morbid thoughts about how this clock had counted down the remaining seconds of Darwin's life and scribbling down my poem.

At that time, I assumed the guide was tactfully leaving the truth of Darwin's health conditions out of the tour because we were a group of children, but I have since learned that the man himself could not have put a name to what ailed him. He lived as a near-invalid for many years, suffering at various times in his life from debilitating headaches, violent heart palpitations, severe gastric upsets, bouts of vomiting and a general anxiety that could not be located in any one body part.

We know from the accounts of others that his symptoms sometimes had a definite physical form, so that at least some of them are verifiable by observation. The headache he had the week before his wedding was so bad that his family considered postponing the ceremony, and a colleague was once astonished upon meeting him after a period of months to find his head so coated in eczema that the great scientist was unrecognisable. But no doctor was ever able to diagnose an underlying cause for these disparate conditions, and in his own writings there is some evidence that Darwin's illness was connected to the anxiety he experienced when he had to deviate from his self-imposed, strict routine of work and rest. The excitement of attending a small dinner party would leave him violently shivering and vomiting for the rest of the night. Darwin channelled his fears into this daily performance of a life ordered by the exertion of the will and he clung to it as the central truth of his existence. Over time, the condition and the supposed cure became indistinguishable.

For six years, Darwin kept what he called *The Diary of Health*, a voluminous daily note of his symptoms. Most of it is filled with notation of flatulence and boils, for which he ingested and applied many Victorian patent remedies of varying toxicity. He also regularly underwent a 'water cure' that involved bathing in and drinking vast quantities of cold water at particular intervals throughout the day. His children's memoirs record that it was a grave sin in the household to interrupt either of these therapeutic interludes or to upset the rhythms of the day as their father had laid them down.

Although undoubtedly unwell, perhaps as a result of his travels to tropical climes as a young man, Darwin also exhibited many of the classic behaviours of the hypochondriac that I find very recognisable. He was fixated on the workings of his own body and obsessive about the methods he had devised to control his fear about them. The baths, the regimented schedule, the reclusiveness – all of it appears designed to keep him from thinking about the abyss that yawned at his feet. His health was a daily drama that he carefully stage-managed. In this, he had less in common with Kant and more with Proust, whose life gradually shrank to his own four walls and then to his bed. The processes Darwin designed that kept him functional took up the majority of his time. At a certain point, a routine meant to prevent the attacks that interfere with life becomes the stuff of life itself.

There have been many posthumous attempts to diagnose Darwin's illnesses. Some experts prefer the theory that it was all a product of his brilliant but overactive mind, a kind of brain fever, while others think that he was a secret arsenic-eater or suffered from a lingering tropical disease. This body of literature is a peculiar subgenre within the literary record of hypochondria, I have discovered – any notable sufferer who made enough of a record of their symptoms attracts this kind of attention. Esteemed and reputable journals like the *British Medical Journal* and *The Lancet* have published many such analyses over the years; John Keats, Katherine Mansfield, Virginia Woolf and many others with both recognisable conditions and hypochondriac tendencies have received this posthumous diagnostic treatment. It's as if we can't bear the absence of a medical explanation for why Woolf experienced intermittent but blinding pain in perfectly good teeth. Hypochondria only has questions, never answers, and that makes us perpetually uneasy.

'Nothing is more punitive than to give a disease a meaning – that meaning being invariably a moralistic one,' Susan Sontag wrote in her 1978 essay *Illness as Metaphor*. As we seek to find meaning in our own experiences, we end up painting that significance onto the disease itself so that over time the illness, and the fear of it, become an embedded part of culture. 'The most truthful way of regarding illness – and the healthiest way of being ill – is one most purified of, most resistant to, metaphoric thinking,' she continues. Illness is a metaphor, or a bundle of metaphors, from which we shape ourselves, but it does us no good. She focuses on tuberculosis and cancer, two conditions that dominated the experience of critical illness in the nineteenth and twentieth centuries. The cultural residue they have left still affects us today; every hypochondriac who fears that they have cancer is, consciously or not, interacting with the metaphorical version of the disease that they have imbibed from a multitude of sources. Everything about the language used to describe cancer is touched by this urge towards metaphor: we say that cancer 'grows' and 'invades', breathing independent life and will into it, rather than the more static 'progresses' or 'develops'. The illness becomes a conscious enemy, putting up a battle, against which someone might win or lose. We cannot help ourselves. Anyone who has shared bad news about a diagnosis knows this; most people cannot stop themselves responding in these terms. *You'll fight it*, they say, before going on to relate the story of a survivor they know, or know of. Perhaps some people find this comforting, and it is always kindly meant, but it makes me want to scream. *Who does this help?*, I silently rage. Piling yet more stories of illness on me just contributes to the feeling that I am slowly being crushed under their weight. The guilt at my less-than-grateful response to these well-meant words is equally crushing, of course.

A defining characteristic of Sontag's writing about illness is how impersonal it is. Anne Boyer, author herself of a memoir about breast cancer, astutely points out that Sontag never uses the words 'I' and 'cancer' in the same sentence. This is part of how she eludes the lure of metaphor, I think: the version of truth that she is trying to convey must come to the reader shorn of autobiography if it is to be resistant to deeper interpretation.

But she was no objective observer, if such a thing even exists. Immediately before writing this essay, Sontag went through two years of extremely invasive chemotherapy for stage four breast cancer that had spread to her lymph nodes, an illness that she recovered from against the odds by, as she put it, 'confounding my doctors' pessimism'. That was the first time she had cancer; she also survived a uterine sarcoma in the 1990s only to be diagnosed again in the early 2000s with the deadly form of leukaemia that ultimately killed her. After her death, her son wrote of her anguished scream when told of this last diagnosis: 'But this means I'm going to die,' she exclaimed, as if this possibility had only just occurred to her.

Despite her careful avoidance of autobiography in *Illness as Metaphor*, readers have long viewed it as a 'personal' text, and rightly so. In a 1987 interview, she explained that her essays are 'mental self-portraits', and that the decision not to tell her own story alongside the critical narrative was a very personal one:

> I felt, out of a combination of shyness, modesty and pride, enormous pride, that I shouldn't mention myself directly, or that I should keep any mention of myself to a minimum. It seemed more elegant and, well, more attractive to me. It was a kind of a pride, as well as timidity, not to bring myself into it, even though I knew there was a considerable autobiographical subtext.

The danger of metaphor is that it can reconfigure our thinking beyond the facts, and lure us into duplicating ideas that are not our own. It encourages fantasy, that there is some moral dimension to illness, for instance. *You don't deserve this*, a well-meaning person will say in the face of a tough diagnosis, as if illness is something that can be avoided by virtue. I was young when I was diagnosed with cancer, a teenager on the brink of adulthood, and I observed how people responded to the idea that the rest of my life might be snatched away before I could experience it. The whole ordeal was somehow laden with so much more meaning because of this accident of timing. There was something angular and uncomfortable about the response to it; people didn't know whether to send me a teddy bear or a book of poetry about death. (Both: the correct answer is both.)

I wonder if the hypochondriac him- or herself is a metaphor, a condensed node of ideas about illness crushed together into one individual. I am pressed between these layers of meaning like a flower preserved between the pages of a book, trapped in narratives about my sickness that have already been written.

One way to resist illness as a metaphor is never to write about it. Or so I thought. I have been running away from opportunities to voice my experiences for years; I once literally hid from a local news reporter in the thick velvet curtains behind the stage at my school hall because I had overheard that he wanted to talk to me about doing a story on 'the promising young student struck down by cancer'. I began my career as a writer in the early 2010s, when the so-called first-person industrial complex was transforming journalism. The internet has a voracious appetite for harrowing personal essays, and paying writers to mine their pasts for horrible experiences with a timely news peg is quicker and cheaper than investing in original reporting. Indeed, it became such a winning formula that a colleague once joked to me that it was possible to ignore the news for a week and then catch up in a few seconds just by reading the list of headlines that all conformed to the writer-centric format 'Why I as an X feel Y about Z'.

The constant pressure to find the personal angle should have

worried me more than it did, I think. The analytics dashboard
for the magazine website where I worked for several years was
like a one-way mirror I could look through into the psyche of
our readers. I sat behind my screen and watched in real time
while the articles, usually by women, in which the authors used
traumatic episodes from their own lives – abortions, sexual
assaults, evictions – as the case studies far outperformed more
traditionally dispassionate writing. There was a thrill in watching the line on the graph bulge and the numbers tick upwards
as more and more readers found a particularly pain-filled article. It felt like a good thing that there was suddenly space for
a wider variety of people to share their experiences, but I now
see how limited an advancement this was. Nobody was giving
these writers the time and resources to write major pieces about
serious subjects; at a time when print was still considered so
much more prestigious, these self-exposing articles tailored to
the rapid churn of the internet almost never crossed over into
physical magazines or newspapers.

Even as I watched this all happening from the wings, I could
never quite shake off the feeling that I would be accelerating
up the career ladder if I could bring myself to mine my life for
trauma to expose for public consumption. And the opportunities were there: I once went to an early meeting about what
would become my first book in which somebody asked me
whether I had lost any close family members in a narratively
convenient way that could 'spice up' the story a bit. In fact,
this is the first time that I have written honestly about being
seriously ill and fearing that I will be ill again. Thinking about
it now, as I am wrist deep in pulling the words out of myself, it
seems peculiar, suspicious even, that I have spent more than a
decade making my living from writing and yet never acknowledged this fundamental part of who I am. My own personal

angle has always been a deception, and the experiences I exposed to view were carefully selected and edited. I've long believed that I am a better editor than I am a writer; I've had a lot of practice on myself.

Telling the story of any illness always involves editing – you leave out the dull, repetitive parts, the embarrassing parts, the most frightening parts. A lack of consistent progress feels irrelevant, and so is easily obscured. At its most extreme, this act of curation can involve saying nothing at all. 'I didn't want to worry you,' a loved one might say when they tell you of a health scare long after the danger has passed. It is easier to describe in the past tense, once the tale has a beginning, a middle and a happy ending. I always think of Fanny Burney, who tried so hard to conceal the horrors of her 1811 mastectomy, performed without any anaesthesia beyond a glass of wine, from her husband. Via her sixteen-year-old son, she arranged for a colleague of her husband's to call him away on 'urgent business' on the day of the operation so that he should not have to witness it. While he was away, seven men held a blindfolded Burney down on her bed while the surgeon worked on her, an experience she later recalled as a kind of torture: 'When the dreadful steel was plunged into the breast – cutting through veins – arteries – flesh – nerves . . . I began a scream that lasted unremittingly during the whole time of the incision,' she wrote. After she had recovered, she feared that garbled rumours of the horrific procedure would reach her family in England, so she wrote out 'the whole history' for her sister in order that she should not be unduly upset. Her husband added a few lines of his own to the letter before it was sent across the Channel – a soldier and a general, he praised Burney's 'sublime courage' and warned his sister-in-law that it had 'almost killed' him to read what his wife had endured during the operation and its aftermath. They were both writing from a place of safety, knowing that the pain which had been endured was now over, that there was a happy ending.

But hypochondria is a plotless story, a deviation from the regular progression of an illness from stage to stage. Without a firm diagnosis for my unreliable symptoms, I am stuck in the first scene of the drama, endlessly looping around the same few lines of dialogue. The compulsion to narrativise this experience is always there, but always thwarted. The comfortable point at which to tell the story never arrives, because everything is always in the present tense. No narrative structure can help those who never get to turn the page on the opening line.

If telling my own story to a doctor, even to myself, has been difficult – full of false starts, reversals, red herrings – the bigger story I am trying to tell about the history of hypochondria itself has proved equally challenging and elusive.

Reconstructing a history for a concept as diffuse and varied as hypochondria is all a matter of tracing reactions. I follow the chains of thought as different minds tackle the same problems down the decades, noting what is retained and what is discarded along the way. I look at the ripples in the water, because most of the time it is impossible to identify the precise moment that the stone was thrown, the moment when the novel idea flashed into being. I want to be able to see the point at which hypochondria ceases to be a physical condition of disordered livers and excess black bile and becomes a problem of the mind, but it is like trying to glimpse the second that a spark jumps across the gap in a circuit: a flash, a crackle, a momentary imprint on the eyelids but nothing that lingers.

At one point, we can come close. In 1766, the eccentric botanist and literary duelist Sir John Hill published *Hypochondriasis*.

A Practical Treatise On The Nature And Cure Of That Disorder; Commonly Called The Hyp And Hypo, which is considered to be the last widely circulated publication to insist that hypochondria was a physical disease. Hill was clearly writing against the prevailing tide of medical opinion, though, because he sees his role as defending the fading primacy of the condition's tangible elements. He says:

> To call the Hypochondriasis a fanciful malady, is ignorant and cruel. It is a real, and a sad disease: an obstruction of the spleen by thickened and distempered blood; extending itself often to the liver, and other parts; and unhappily in England very frequent: physick scarce knows one more fertile in ill; or more difficult of cure.

He does, however, admit that there are some mental elements that aggravate the symptoms of this spleen blockage. Emotional turmoil, such as that caused by grief and love, can trigger an attack. He also suggests that 'indolence and inactivity are oftenest at the root', although it has sometimes also been caused by too much activity. Too much reading and studying can bring it on, not so much because of the mental strain but because of 'the stooping posture of the body, which most men use, though none should use it, in writing and in reading'. Compressing the torso is more likely to injure the organs of the hypochondriac region and bring on hypochondria. But if you are unlucky enough to catch it, Hill has a cure for you. Spleenwort, which grows as a small evergreen fern, when taken as a powder or tincture can gradually dissolve the blockage in the spleen that causes hypochondria. Relief soon follows, as 'the patient feels the happy change that is growing in his constitution' thanks to the removal of this physical obstacle to health. Fortunately, Hill is available to prepare this medicine for you, should you need it.

It should be said that Hill is a somewhat dubious source, although a fascinating character. He had a long and varied career, which included practising as an apothecary and a quack doctor, feuding at length with Henry Fielding and David Garrick in the London press, and falsely taking credit for one of the most popular cookery books of the eighteenth century. His biographer describes his life as 'a series of paradoxes without coherence' and notes that although Hill made useful scientific contributions to the botanical classification of vegetables, he was above all a provocateur who started a famous feud with the Royal Society about the biological viability of immaculate conception after they refused to elect him as a fellow.

Hill was a contrarian, then, so it follows that he would be the last to dig his heels in for the fundamentally physical nature of hypochondria. Even if he was not making any advance in the medical understanding of the condition, he was at least adept at capturing the contemporary fascination with it. The lengthy subtitle of his book points to the fact that this had become a major topic of discourse for the chattering classes of the eighteenth century. The word 'hypochondria' was uttered so often that it was abbreviated to 'hyp' or 'hypo' for ease of conversational flow and no doubt to save printing ink. Thirty-five years before Hill's treatise was published, 'hyp' was already such a common contraction that two popular poems about hypochondria published in the same year used it in their titles. In 1731, both William Somervile's 'The Hyp: a Burlesque Poem in Five Cantos' and Tim Scrubb's 'A Rod for the Hyp-Doctor' appeared. And it is possible that a version of this contracted form of the word survives in English usage today. There is a theory that the idiom 'you give me the pip', meaning 'you annoy me', was originally a corruption of 'you give me the hyp'. As a retort it is quite satisfying: 'you make me feel like I have a melancholy, angsty, nebulous disease' is a rare insult. The contraction was certainly popular among the literati. When Alexander Pope died in 1744, he declared to his friend Joseph Spence as he neared his end that 'I never was hippish in my whole life', and nearly eighty years later Byron wrote in his diary that he was 'rather in low spirits – certainly hippish – liver touched – will take a dose of salts'.

In 1822, the year after Byron made this entry, a French doctor specialising in mental disorders named Jean-Pierre Falret published a pivotal book titled *De l'Hypochondrie et du suicide*, in which he states absolutely that hypochondria was an entirely mental condition, part of the overarching *folie* or 'madness' that serves as the contemporary term for mental health disorders. 'Moral and intellectual causes are, without contradiction, the most usual causes of hypochondria,' he writes. He lists many common symptoms that he had observed in his patients: insomnia, chest pains, a ringing in the ears, digestive problems, an excessive fixation on their bodily symptoms and health, a disproportionate interest in medical texts and news, and imaginary symptoms. 'I saw a lady who, by sight, judged that her skin was scaly like that of a carp, but at the same instant she could rectify her judgment by touch,' he records. Her skin was smooth, he is suggesting, but she disbelieves the evidence of her own senses and those of the doctor in favour of the impression she has formed in her mind – an example of what later will be termed a 'medically unexplained symptom'. Falret is gracious towards those who have come before him with their mistaken beliefs about the organs of the hypochondriac region as being the cause of their maladies, attributing this error to two fundamental inaccuracies. Firstly, his predecessors did not know about the brain's role at the centre of a nervous system that governs sensation in the body, he says, and secondly, they came to hypochondria with the preconceived notions of humoral theory, so of course they found digestive symptoms to support their ideas.

Falret is remembered now for his prescient identification of what he called *la folie circulaire* – known today as bipolar disorder – but his role in the history of hypochondria cannot be underestimated. Somewhere in the murky decades between John Hill's treatise in 1766 and Falret's work in 1822 the tide of medical opinion turned, and hypochondria became generally accepted as a condition of the mind. But it was Falret who finally separated it from millennia of association with liver, spleen and intestines. The idea of the soul, the meaningful consciousness of a person, as a wild animal chained to the liver was at last displaced by a new conception of identity and awareness tied to the brain. Although these organs (as well as others) might exhibit the effects of hypochondria, they were no longer the centre or its cause. From now on, it was the mind that controlled the body's experiences and sensations, not the other way around. His work paved the way for the next century of advances in the understanding of how a condition that presented in the body could reside in the mind, as the understanding and treatment of mental illness moved from asylums to First World War convalescent hospitals to psychiatrists' consulting rooms.

The rise of psychoanalysis at the end of the nineteenth century left hypochondria in a strangely isolated position. Early psychologists like Jean-Martin Charcot and then Pierre Janet in France, and William James in America were eagerly exploring the potential for past memories to create present-day mental obstacles. Janet wrote that 'certain happenings would leave indelible and distressing memories – memories to which the sufferer was continually returning, and by which he was tormented by day and by night'. The implications of this for mental illness, especially when later combined with Josef Breuer's early experiments with a 'talking cure' for hysteria, were profound, but nobody was keen to try to fit hypochondria into this new paradigm. Charcot's work at the Salpêtrière teaching hospital in Paris had once more separated hysteria from hypochondria, with the former confirmed as a purely mental illness – the 'epitome of neurosis' – and the latter left ambiguous and confused. The gender separation of the two conditions was debunked too, with Charcot presenting several cases of what he called 'traumatic male hysteria' that finally put paid to the idea there was something inherently female about the condition. The exciting progress at this time was in the field of mental distress and neurosis; indeed, this had become fashionable in a way that hypochondria had been in the early eighteenth century. The preoccupation with the power of the unconscious mind that Sigmund Freud ushered in entrenched the idea that there were two distinct kinds of health problem: physical diseases and mental illnesses. Hypochondria was at once both and neither: a mental condition with physical manifestations. Unlike with hysteria, no link to past memories or trauma was discerned for hypochondria.

Freud had a lot less to say about hypochondria than we might assume; it was not at all a helpful asset to his developing theories about the mind. He wrote to his friend the German otolaryngologist Wilhelm Fliess in November 1887 about his difficulty in determining if a patient, Mrs A, was suffering from a neurosis or the onset of a 'systemic disease' like multiple sclerosis. 'In neurasthenia the hypochondriacal alteration, the anxiety psychosis, is never missing and, whether denied or admitted, betrays itself by a profusion of newly emerging sensations, that is, by paresthesias,' he declared. Mrs A had neither the anxiety nor the tingling and numbness (known as paraesthesia, or 'pins and needles') that Freud seemingly considered essential to hypochondria, and so her problems must lie elsewhere. By 1895, Freud had made the – to us, unsurprising, given the general direction of his work – link between hypochondria and sexual dysfunction, telling Fliess that the hypochondriac typically 'will not admit to himself that [his illness] arises from his sexual life'. His idea was developed further in a paper one of his students, Isidor Sadger, gave to the Vienna Psychoanalytic Society in May 1911. 'Persons with a traumatic neurosis become hypochondriacs in that, having been rejected in their demands on all sides, they throw their libido onto their own illness. In this sense, hypochondria is the state of being in love with one's own illness,' Sadger declared, while Freud looked on from the audience. But nothing is settled: two years before, Freud had said during a discussion of his work on hysteria and psychoneuroses at the Vienna Psychoanalytic Society that one had 'to admit frankly, for example, that the position of hypochondria is still suspended in darkness'. Later, he associated it with narcissism and the idea that the bond between libido and ego becomes stronger through a shared investment in the region of the body that is perceived as diseased – a kind of sick self-love.

Crucially, though, Freud decided that hypochondria is one of three 'pure forms of true neurosis' with a physical basis as opposed to a psychoneurosis, in which the symptoms are drawn from the libido.

The symptoms of an actual neurosis – headache, sensation of pain, an irritable condition of some organ, the weakening or inhibition of some function – have no 'meaning,' no signification in the mind. Not merely are they manifested principally in the body, as also happens, for instance with hysterical symptoms, but they are in themselves purely and simply physical processes; they arise without any of the complicated mental mechanisms we have been learning about.

This lack of meaning, of narrative significance, leads to the conclusion that hypochondria cannot be treated with analysis in the way that the true neuroses can. It came to be thought of as 'unanalysable' and was thus of no interest to the burgeoning field of psychoanalysis.

There is a hint though, in a letter to Fliess in 1894, that Freud was concerned about his own propensity towards hypochondria. He lays out his case history for his friend, saying that he has not been well and begging for an expert opinion. The tone of the letter is uncharacteristically chaotic and a little panicked. On Fliess's advice, he gave up smoking for seven weeks, he says, but found that it left him 'completely incapable of working, a beaten man', and that having seen a couple of patients with similar symptoms during this period who have never smoked, he decides to start again. This improves matters somewhat – three cigars a day, apparently, is enough to make him feel able to work again – but he still is not well. He has attacks of heart palpitations and an irregular pulse, mostly after lunch, as well as 'stabbing pains, a feeling of oppression, and burning sensations'. He is still sleeping well, but he feels 'aged, sluggish, not healthy'.

The most hypochondria-like feature of his illness, though, is his fixation on the vagueness of it all. 'What tortures me is the uncertainty about what to make of the story. It would embarrass me to suggest a hypochondriacal evaluation, but I have no criteria by which to decide this,' he says. He has consulted his friend the physician Josef Breuer, who to Freud's disgust is treating him 'like a patient'. He sounds just like me in the grip of a hypochondriacal tantrum: the doctor is not listening to him, he is just telling him what he wants to hear, he is not seeing him regularly enough, and he never gives straight answers to questions. 'I would be endlessly obliged to you, though, if you were to give me a definite explanation, since I secretly believe that you know precisely what it is,' he concludes his letter to his friend, sounding desperate. Subsequent letters suggest that Fliess's prescription was to give up cigars again, which Freud grudgingly did, and then ten months later he reports feeling 'quite unbelievably well' after 'a cocainization of the left nostril'. Fliess was a proponent of the now thoroughly debunked theory that the nose acted as a microcosm of the body, and that applying cocaine to the correct part of the nostril could cure the corresponding ailment elsewhere in the body; he also once published a paper titled 'The Relation between the Nose and the Female Sexual Organs'. Freud seems to have been an enthusiastic test subject of this method, and as is so commonly the case, doing something about his nebulous feelings of sickness seems to have allayed both his symptoms and his fears that he would require that embarrassing 'hypochondriacal evaluation'. That, and the energising effect of regular bumps of cocaine, no doubt.

It is surprising that Freud did not find a bigger place for hypochondria in his work because it seems to me that, at its simplest, hypochondria is a fear of death. Or perhaps it is more accurate to call it *fear* of the fear of death. In the worst moments of uncertainty, the idea of being given a terminal diagnosis and a remaining period of time to live is not the most terrifying outcome. Those who live relatively anxiety-free lives will not understand this at all, but there is a certain – very strange – satisfaction to be gained from seeing the worst-case scenario come true. At least it would be solid information, from which a plan could be made for the time that is left. Not knowing is constantly living on the edge of a precipice, braced for the fall but never actually falling off. It is existing in perpetual limbo, never being sure if tomorrow will come in the same way that today did. The present is ruined for fear of what the future might bring.

In this sense, hypochondria is merely the human condition with the comforting fictions stripped away. Whether we choose to think about it all the time or not, we are all just one freak accident away from the end. It all gets mawkish very quickly: every goodbye could be the last goodbye; every Christmas could be the last Christmas; every sunset could be the final sunset. We have all heard the stories about outwardly healthy marathon-running people who pass away far too young, or the sudden calamities that should never have happened but sadly do. This morbid spiralling makes functioning during day-to-day life impossible, of course, but it is not founded on completely baseless speculation. For all that humanity has built systems and precautions to reduce the likelihood of random mortality, we can't ever filter it out completely. Life, even in its most sheltered, privileged form, is far more precarious than we think it is. A hypochondriac is someone who is just a little more aware of this than the average person, we might say. This is the fundamental irony of hypochondria, in fact. My symptoms might be undetectable and my fears baseless, but something will get me in the end, regardless.

Is an exaggerated awareness of one's own mortality a cause of hypochondria, or a symptom of it? Experts agree that 'the excessive fear of death seems to be one of the fundamental, underlying characteristics of hypochondriasis', and studies measuring the attitudes towards death of those with high levels of health anxiety support this view, but there is little consensus on which comes first. There are theories, too, about hypochondria being a psychological response to the feeling of powerlessness that comes with exposure to the myriad threats to human life, or a natural accompaniment to an awareness of the meaninglessness of existence. The death of a loved one is often the trigger for the onset of hypochondria for this reason; if they were taken, the bereaved person reasons, why not me too? A common theme among the self-described hypochondriacs I have spoken to over the last several years has been a fixation on the age at which a close friend or relative has died, even if there is nothing to suggest that there are any shared health conditions or risk factors. 'How could I make it past thirty-seven when she didn't?' said one person who had lost an older sister.

Even when you do live with this heightened awareness of mortality, its confirmation can come as a shock. When I was about halfway through writing this book, I had just such an experience: a routine screening for a potential side effect of the radiation treatment I'd had for my blood cancer turned up something worthy of further investigation, and it sent me into a vertiginous emotional decline. The letter's wording was vague – we need to do further tests, it said, and we can't tell you any more until we have – and the section where there should have been resources for further information just had the place-holder text '<insert helpline number here>' printed on it. When I later showed this to the doctor in an attempt to communicate how much this letter had destabilised me mentally and to suggest that perhaps they should include more information for patients up front, she laughed and took a picture of the printing error to show her colleagues. As a method of reassurance, I would not recommend this.

The appointment was scheduled for two weeks later, and in fact I ended up needing two further rounds of tests over the next several months before the suspicious cells were finally deemed harmless. This cluster, which had looked so odd on an MRI scan, had likely been there for years, the doctor said. But once I was aware of it, nothing felt the same, even though it was actually the same. I was just as much in danger as I had been the day before receiving the letter, I just hadn't known about it. Throughout the whole process, I experienced what I can only describe as a sharpening of perspective. The world looked brighter to me somehow, like a photograph with the saturation level turned right up. I experienced the usual falling dominos of catastrophisation: what if I was too ill to work, what if I couldn't take the pain, what if my dog missed me when I died, what if nobody came to my funeral, what if my husband met someone else after I was gone, what if he didn't, what if, what if, what if? Once I waded through the worst of this in the first forty-eight hours, though, a sense of peace settled on me that I initially found extremely disturbing, and then addictive. Nothing seemed to matter anymore, at least in comparison to the fate that awaited me. The normal niggles of everyday life just vanished from view. I wanted to bottle this feeling, to live like this all the time, in a state of being where frustrating customer helplines and public transport delays did not affect me at all because they were not bad medical news. I tried telling friends about this mortality-induced euphoria, but soon stopped after a few baffled, even offended, reactions. It was hard to convey how I could feel so completely terrified and utterly content at the same time. And of course, the feeling did not last. As the immediate danger receded, so did my heightened sense of existence as something fleeting and fragile and precious. My days were still numbered – as they always have been – but I could not recapture the serenity that had come with the knowledge that the number was lower than expected.

The most common treatment that someone seeking help with health anxiety will be offered is cognitive behavioural therapy (CBT). This is a talking therapy that, in its simplest form, seeks to alter both the way a patient thinks and how they behave when presented with a scenario they find distressing. In the case of hypochondria specifically, the recommended protocol focuses on the particular patterns of thought and behaviour that the person regularly engages in and works on altering them so as to alleviate their suffering.

The part about CBT that I find especially intriguing is the emphasis it places on confronting, rather than avoiding, uncomfortable thoughts and habits. So much of hypochondria for me is about dissociation, being the brain in the jar who can't feel what is happening in her body, that the notion of doing the opposite of what my instincts want is quite perplexing. To try to understand this apparently contradictory approach further, I consulted Dr Becky Spelman, a CBT therapist of two decades' experience with health anxiety clients, whose calm exterior, I soon realised, concealed a steely and creative brain when it came to devising exercises for her hypochondriac patients.

'Our natural instinct is avoid, avoid and protect ourselves. Don't feel anxious,' she said. 'We get the relief that we need from whatever the behaviour is, whether it's googling a symptom or seeking reassurance from a friend, and then we don't break the cycle.'

Part of the collaboration between patient and therapist

involves inventing exercises that gently ramp up towards confronting the primary source of the anxiety. For hypochondriacs, an important one can be simply to do nothing when the urge to check a symptom rears its head. As someone who has literally sat on her hands before to stop herself poking a suspected lump, I know how difficult inaction can be at these times. As Spelman explains, 'It's hard to believe in those moments of high anxiety that actually not doing anything is absolutely fine. The mind plays tricks on us and says, oh, but what if it's not health anxiety on this occasion? What if it really is the illness? Or maybe just one last check and then I'll get the reassurance I need. And of course, that makes someone feel better in the short term, but then they get stuck in the cycle again.'

CBT involves running, metaphorically, towards the danger that the mind wants so desperately to flee. And you have to do it over and over again, Spelman says, to combat the temptation to go back to the old ways. If someone had a particular fear of germs and getting sick, for instance, their therapist might set them the task of taking public transport, and then 'touching their shoe and licking their palm'. 'I'd ask them to make a prediction too,' she explains. 'Do they think that that will make them ill in a week's time? You want to think about how can we actually make them more anxious than they would normally be in relation to their health anxiety.'

This kind of desensitisation goes together with a reframing of thought as something that can be governed, rather than just experienced. Even if the hypochondriacal thoughts feel automated, like they are out of our control, CBT teaches techniques for interacting with them, even reasoning with them, before discarding them if they are unhelpful. For clients who have a serious illness as well as health anxiety this can be especially important; Spelman cites the example of someone with diagnosed diabetes who fixates on their glucose monitor to the extent that it interferes with their daily life. 'It's about helping them realise what is actually the health anxiety side of it and what is the diabetes. The emotional reaction is going to be irrational and not very helpful to managing their condition.' Showing someone that their behaviour is excessive and illogical, or teaching them the difference between the symptoms of anxiety and those of a heart attack, say, can help them to break out of the unhelpful patterns that much more quickly.

'A good question to ask is "What is the worst thing that could happen?"' Spelman concludes. Confronting the mortality that hypochondria makes so very present and terrifying is intrinsic to finding any kind of relief through this method.

Even if contemplating my inevitable death is the last thing I want to do when my anxiety levels are rising, it is in art, I think, where we grapple best with the truncated nature of our existence, where the contradictory fears of death and hypochondria best find expression. I find myself drawn to works that slyly wink at the notion of mortality, echoing that black comedy inherent to hypochondria. I particularly like the Salvador Dalí portrait titled *In Voluptas Mors*, in which photographer Philippe Halsman captured the Spanish artist in profile in the foreground, wearing a top hat and looking with wide, startled eyes across the frame. In the background, dominating the whole picture, is an arrangement of seven nude female figures that, when glanced at quickly, looks like a skull with dark sunken eye sockets between bones formed of white exposed flesh. When the viewer focuses in on the skull, the details of the women's poses break the illusion – we can see how two pairs of feet hang down into a void to suggest teeth and the artful backbend of one flexible woman across the top of a black-draped structure forms the brow. The title of the picture roughly translates as 'voluptuous death', suggesting that we are supposed to find something titillating in the presentation of so much nakedness on film. In fact, I find that the closer I look at the models, the better the picture functions as a kind of wry *memento mori*. The woman who forms the eye sockets at the centre of the composition is posed with arms outstretched, almost Christ-like, and her face is tilted upwards as if in exhortation. Her ribs are visible on the sides of her torso and there is very little that is alluring about her, for all that her breasts are exposed. In the picture, her whole body is standing in for bone, and I can see her bones beneath her skin.

There is a fable from the Babylonian Empire, in the second millennium BCE, that I think about a lot in relation to the hypochondriac's fear of death too. Usually titled 'When Death Came to Baghdad' or 'Appointment in Samarra', it has been variously adapted in the Jewish and Muslim literary traditions for hundreds of years, and was then retold by W. Somerset Maugham in the mid-twentieth century. In it, a servant is sent to market and returns in terror to his master with a tale of having been threatened by the figure of Death in Baghdad's crowded marketplace. The servant begs, and is granted, permission to take one of his master's horses and flee to Samarra, a stronghold to the north of the city. Later in the day, when the master goes to market himself and meets Death there disguised as an old woman, he asks him why he threatened his servant. The response comes, in Maugham's version: 'It was only an expression of surprise. I was astonished to see him in Baghdad, for I had an appointment with him tonight in Samarra.' There is no escaping our ultimate fate, and attempting to do so only results in a lot of wasted energy. If only such a rationale could free a hypochondriac from their fears.

I find these themes developed in the most unexpected of places. The 2020 teen comedy film *Spontaneous*, which follows the fortunes of a class at an American high school after students start spontaneously exploding, is an unlikely hypochondria text. And yet it fits perfectly: those teenagers who have not yet 'popped like a zit' in a wave of dark red gore become terrified that they will be next. The adults around them scramble to construct theories about why some kids liquify and others don't, and what the underlying cause of it all might be. The film's protagonists Mara and Dylan crack jokes as they are hustled first into an isolation ward, and then into separate plastic bubbles so that this mysteriously traceless affliction cannot spread any further than it already has. Eventually, though, the relentless horror and fear gets to Mara; she ends up lying on the grass, sobbing. 'I don't know what to do with my body, it feels like I'm dying, I'm so scared all the time,' she wails. Dylan's grieving mother, stretched out next to her, gives her a gentle but firm pep talk about how fear and death are unrelated; worrying that something bad will happen will not prevent it from happening. 'Do you want to come over for dinner next week?' she concludes, matter-of-factly. There is nothing to do but keep going, she is implying. The ground may open up and swallow you any moment, or your flesh may somehow splatter into the air, but those are only more dramatic versions of what we all face anyway.

Nobody dreaded death more poetically, and more constantly, than Philip Larkin. A long-term hypochondriac, he was forever convinced that his life was about to end, and that he had wasted it. 'Life is first boredom, then fear. / Whether or not we use it, it goes,' he wrote in one of his most famous poems, which plumbs the depths of his disillusionment. From earliest childhood he had poor eyesight, and almost as soon as he learned to speak he had a stammer. He was a clumsy child who grew into a tall and ungainly man, who always looked older and sadder than his years. The American poet Robert Lowell met him in 1973, when he was fifty years old, and afterwards wrote to his friend Elizabeth Bishop that Larkin looked older than T. S. Eliot, who had been born over forty years before him. Larkin's hypochondria was engendered in part by his unhappy home life: his parents had met by chance at a holiday resort on the Welsh coast and got engaged three days later, and by the time Philip came along they were well entrenched in their combative attitudes to each other. Sydney Larkin was domineering and Eva was timid and compliant. Their home was not overtly violent, but Larkin grew up in what his biographer Andrew Motion has described as an atmosphere of 'clenched irritation', with the sense that any second the suppressed anger could boil over into rage.

Larkin's father encouraged his son's nascent interest in literature as a teenager, but they were not close. Sydney – an accountant for the city council – was a male chauvinist, according to his secretary, and an ardent and long-time admirer of Hitler and the Nazis. He thought very highly of Germany under the Nazis, carried on an enthusiastic correspondence with Hjalmar Schacht, Hitler's Minister of Economics from 1934 to 1937, and had to be ordered to take down the Nazi regalia decorating his office at Coventry City Hall when Britain declared war on Germany in 1939. In later life, Philip told a friend that his father had been present at several Nuremberg rallies in the 1930s and had a figurine of Hitler on the mantelpiece that performed the Nazi salute when you touched a button. He was neither warm nor sympathetic, and he disapproved of many of Larkin's school friends to the point where his son lived a fairly isolated existence as a teenager. According to Philip's later account, his mother was a whining, self-pitying creature who was constantly suspicious that she was being lied to by her autocratic husband and her silent son. Once, she leapt up from the breakfast table suddenly and announced that she would be committing suicide. She was tenacious about household routines, and imprinted upon Larkin the idea that any deviation from the norm was something to be very alarmed about. The smallness and misery of the life she wove about herself both attracted and repelled him. It became his poetic milieu – 'Deprivation is to me what daffodils were to Wordsworth,' he once said – but it also made him yearn for an escape he never quite achieved. His mother was a burden to him, but one that he clutched close. He wrote to her twice a week for thirty-five years, beginning when he left home at eighteen to go to university, and visited her often.

In 1955, now working as a librarian at the University of Hull, he visited his mother in the Midlands for Christmas and found her unwell with something that her doctor could not diagnose. She spent a month in hospital convalescing, during which time Larkin was simultaneously terrified that she would die and also that she would recover and continue to be a burden to him. As soon as she was on the mend, his own health suddenly went downhill, as if he had caught whatever nebulous sickness was plaguing her. He had an X-ray for a suspected stomach ulcer and tortured himself with ideas of the deadly cancer that would soon be revealed, but was told by his doctor that there was nothing to worry about. From this experience, though, Larkin came away with a fear of his throat becoming constricted or blocked. It became his habit before every meal to drink large glasses of water so as to open his throat sufficiently to swallow food – a practice that recalls the 'water cures' enjoyed by

Darwin and other hypochondriacs the century before. He felt himself always tethered to his mother's wellbeing: ten years later he wrote to his lover Monica Jones of his mother that 'I suppose I shall become free at sixty, three years before cancer starts,' but in fact Eva lived until 1977, when Larkin was fifty-five, dying in her sleep at the age of ninety-one, and he had seven years before he was diagnosed with cancer.

Larkin's hypochondria became more acute at times of great emotional turmoil, his fear over his mother's health being just one instance. In 1961, he collapsed at work during a meeting of the library committee and had to be carried 'unconscious and incontinent' to an ambulance. Once he came to in the hospital, he tried very hard to convince the doctors that the problem had been caused by the combination of a too-tight shirt collar and wearing glasses with the wrong prescription, but they kept him in for observation and further tests. He quickly descended into spiralling anxiety about what might be wrong with him, unable now to separate the issues that had originally caused his collapse from his terror at being in the hospital. He wrote long, incoherent letters to Monica, documenting his escalating panic:

> This place has begun to depress me: I feel frightfully alone and uncared for. Is all this a sort of breakdown? Should I 'try to buck up', and all that? It's not just feeling depressed: I feel depressed because my head still feels wrong: it isn't pain of any kind, but a kind of swimming giddiness that undermines everything I do, and makes it impossible for me to *enjoy* doing anything. And this in turn worries me and gives me a central apprehensiveness in the chest.

He indulges in long diagnostic speculations too, wondering if he in fact has two illnesses, not one, that are conspiring to cause his disparate symptoms. He dreads X-rays and blood tests, even though those are the tools that will enable the doctors to give him more information about his condition, and describes himself as being 'caught up in another backwash of apprehension' every time he thinks about what might be revealed to him. A junior doctor tells him that whatever ails him, it is 'nothing common', and this both cheers and daunts him – the snobbish part of him being delighted that he is proving to be a patient worthy of intellectual enquiry, the hypochondriac portion now terrified that he will end up in a London brain clinic being operated on for some rare malady. He is honest with Monica about what truly ails him: 'Of course the real trouble is I'm rigid with funk.' His symptoms included vision problems, sweating, flu-like issues, sore bowels, a coated tongue, loss of appetite and 'being aware of my right eye', but his most acute sensation was fear. 'I'm afraid I'm seriously ill, & really this is all that's in my mind, and nobody can give me any comfort,' he wrote.

In his biography, Andrew Motion suggests it is strange that nobody at the hospital or indeed afterwards investigated whether there was a psychological component to Larkin's sudden illness. In the months before his collapse, he had begun a romantic relationship with a colleague, Maeve Brennan, in addition to his long-standing affair with Monica. A few weeks before his hospitalisation, Monica had discovered his feelings for another woman, and the state of his emotional life was miserable and tense. 'He hadn't been able to deal with the drama any more; he had blacked out,' Motion suggests. This matches the medical evidence: after exhaustive investigations, the Hull doctors could find nothing discernible wrong with him. He spent time in a London clinic, and was eventually diagnosed by an eminent neurosurgeon with 'epilepsy of late onset with no positive evidence of an organic cause'. He was then discharged to resume his life, and never had another recurrence of the same illness.

A few weeks before his hospitalisation, he had written 'Ambulances', a poem about the inevitability of death. 'They come to rest at any kerb: / All streets in time are visited,' the first stanza concludes. Like Robert Burton, Larkin had long been fixated on the date of his own death. He was obsessed with the idea that he would die at the same age as his father, sixty-three, and his own trip to the hospital in an ambulance appears to have confirmed to him that he was correct in this belief. He wrote to Maeve while he was convalescing that 'I feel rather depressed and unwilling to resume a life which hasn't got much to recommend it – I mean it was a blind alley sort of existence, leading nowhere but THE GRAVE'. That's his capitalisation. The grave overshadows all else.

In a review that he wrote of a book about Thomas Hardy, Larkin attempted to use the index as a way of unravelling the different facets of his subject's character. He read down the list: 'Hypochondria, self-absorption, stinginess, luxuriating in misery, selfishness, inhospitality, susceptibility to young women, mother-fixation.' If he read himself in those words too, Larkin did not say so, but the accuracy of the character sketch is uncanny. Hardy's letters are also full of complaints about his health: he worried about his rheumatism, he suffered from chills upon the liver, and at one point complained of the 'English cholera', without explaining what that really was. Larkin was a great admirer of Hardy and occasionally drew parallels between them himself – when his mother died at the age of ninety-one, he remarked that Hardy's mother had passed away at the same age.

The hardest part of Larkin's hypochondria to grapple with is that he was, in several ways, proved correct in his fears. Having worried about a feeling of constriction in his throat for decades, in 1985 it was cancer of the oesophagus that eventually laid him low, a brutal diagnosis that required an operation to remove the infected tissue in an attempt to stem the tide of metastasising cells that had already spread through his body. He struggled on for four months in increasingly ill health, falling down a lot and experiencing severe pain. Eventually he was readmitted to hospital in November of that year, and died four days later. His last words, as he clutched the hand of the nurse who sat with him were 'I am going to the inevitable.' After a lifetime of battling against his own mortality, of dreading illness and flinching away from the brevity of his existence, he seems to have accepted it at the end. He was sixty-three years old when he died. Chance, or premonition? The hypochondriac's eternal dilemma: am I worrying over nothing, and is my worrying in fact making my worries come true? For all his clean, spare poetry about desolation and decay, this is the knotted, tangled riddle with which Larkin left us.

As Larkin's example shows, health concerns and fear of death can induce a feeling of profound and terrifying powerlessness. But Jane Austen had a different take on this. In her work, hypochondria – or at least the ostentatious display of hypochondriac behaviour – can be a way of wielding power, especially in intimate relationships. Her novels are densely populated by hypochondriacs; on a per-novel basis, she surely outpaces any other writer in the English language. The imaginary illnesses of *Emma*'s Mr Woodhouse and Mrs Churchill, *Persuasion*'s Mary Musgrove, *Mansfield Park*'s Lady Bertram, *Pride and Prejudice*'s Mrs Bennet and Marianne from *Sense and Sensibility* are woven tightly into the social fabric of her books. They are not just described for comic effect – although Austen certainly does enjoy highlighting the absurdity of this condition – but examined for what they reveal about the attachments and tensions between the characters. She is especially interested in unexpressed social tension and how the hypochondriac can wield their fears as a weapon to make sure that everyone around them concurs with their wishes.

Austen's novels are littered with invalids, cases of nerves, fainting fits, chronic fatigue and colds that require the patient to retire immediately to bed and be seen by a doctor daily. She has plenty of characters who understand the social advantage to be gained in a well-pitched performance of being unwell too: think of Mrs Bennet in *Pride and Prejudice* sending Jane to Netherfield on horseback rather than in a carriage so she might catch a cold and therefore spend more time with Mr Bingley, or Harriet Smith in *Emma* spraining an ankle and being deftly manoeuvred into the arms of Frank Churchill for the rest of the walk. Austen's light touch belies the cunning with which she makes sure the reader knows which illnesses are worth taking seriously: Jane's time in bed at Netherfield is never presented as anything other than genuine, whereas we are constantly encouraged not to believe in Mrs Bennet's pain. 'She was a woman of mean understanding, little information, and uncertain temper. When she was discontented she fancied herself nervous,' she tells us. Her faults are moral, not physical. In Elizabeth Bennet, the book has a heroine of quick wit and great intelligence, which is contrasted unfavourably with the shamefully hysterical behaviour of her not at all clever mother, who uses her attacks to keep her family's wishes subordinate to her own. For instance:

Tell Mr Bennet what a dreadful state I am in, – that I am frightened out of my wits; and have such tremblings, such flutterings, all over me, such spasms in my side, and pains in my head, and such beatings at heart, that I can get no rest by night nor by day.

She is roundly ridiculed for this, both by the narratorial voice of the novel and her own husband, who mocks her with a parody of her own behaviour:

It gives such an elegance to misfortune! Another day I will do the same; I will sit in my library, in my nightcap and powdering gown, and give as much trouble as I can.

Mr Woodhouse, father of the heroine of *Emma*, also 'fancies himself nervous' – he is, we are told, a nervous man whose 'spirits required support'. He is a man, though, and a rich one at that, so those around him pander to him rather than ridicule him. 'His wobbly spirits are supported by almost everyone with whom he comes in contact: an army of servants; his neighbours; his personal apothecary; and most of all Emma, his devoted daughter'. He is free of gendered notions of hysteria or sensibility, although his querulous demands that all draughts be immediately quenched and no door ever slammed don't strike the modern-day reader as especially rational or justified. He also uses his anxiety about his health as a means of control, binding his daughter to him permanently in the interests of keeping his household and his habits exactly the same and preventing her from achieving any kind of independent life. His apothecary, Mr Perry, is constantly referred to and quoted by Mr Woodhouse and others, but never speaks himself – a way for Austen to emphasise Perry's true role in their lives, not as a provider of expertise or technical prowess, but rather a source of reassurance, a crutch for the hypochondriac. Deborah Levy brings this dynamic into the twenty-first century in her 2016 novel *Hot Milk*, in which a daughter, Sofia, accompanies her perpetually ailing mother, Rose, to a dubious and highly expensive clinic in Spain for a 'cure'. The two are bound together by the perpetual uncertainty of Rose's health – will she be able to walk today, or not? – and Sofia even sometimes experiences sympathy pains prompted by her mother's unreliable symptoms. Her ability to focus, and indeed her whole life, begins to disintegrate thanks to the influence of Rose's fragmentary health problems.

Austen's repeated use of hypochondria as a means of parental control – in *Emma*, Frank Churchill's rich aunt is also constantly summoning him to her bedside, seemingly just for the sake of making him jump when she calls – brings to mind a rare psychological disorder known as factitious disorder imposed on another (FDIA), previously called Munchausen syndrome by proxy. It affects caregivers, often to very young children, and involves deliberately neglecting or even making the child sick so as to be able to seek medical assistance and receive attention. Although this horrifying form of abuse is not hypochondria, it does have some interesting parallels with the kind of power dynamics that Austen highlights in association with the condition.

Austen's hypochondriacs are not all so grim, however. In *Persuasion*, Anne Elliot's sister Mary Musgrove is, on the surface, a comic hypochondriac; everyone seems aware of her foibles and humours them with varying degrees of kindness. But beneath this is a much sadder picture, of a young woman who knows that she was her husband's second choice for a wife, who grew up in the knowledge that her two older sisters were each the preferred child of one parent, who feels overlooked and ignored by her exuberant in-laws, and who finds the sensation of being constantly tolerated rather than liked extremely depressing. Unfortunately, her chosen method for turning attention back on herself is to complain loudly and long about physical ailments that come and go as her mood requires, which in turn makes her even more isolated as other characters do their best to give her and her complaints a wide berth. Mary is also an expert in whining, and can always be relied upon to do it in such a way as to 'raise the emotional temperature of any dialogue'. She speaks always in extremes, because nothing can be allowed to top her suffering as the centre of attention: 'My sore throats, you know, are always worse than anybody's'; 'I began to think I should never see you. I am so ill I can hardly speak.' Her health is one weapon in the arsenal she deploys to get what she wants. She vocalises her unhappiness constantly, using her imaginary health issues as the medium to do so. Anne, meanwhile, buries her unhappiness and never speaks of it to anybody – which is ultimately rewarded by the novel's happy resolution in her favour, leaving no doubt as to which approach Austen herself endorses.

There was a particular reason why Jane Austen was so interested in the ripple effect that a committed hypochondriac could cause within a family: she had personal experience of it. Her mother, Cassandra Leigh Austen, suffered throughout her life with ailments that Jane felt were 'chiefly in her head'. Mrs Austen's symptoms seemed to vary according to mood and season; at one point she had 'an asthma, a dropsy, water in her chest, and a liver disorder' and later on in her life she suffered from terrible biliousness. She has been described by critics as 'a lifelong hypochondriac' of the kind who always has the excuse of their health to prevent them doing anything unpleasant, but can stage a miraculous recovery when a congenial activity is proposed. Jane often sounds peevish and frustrated when she wrote to relatives about her mother's perpetual ailments: in one missive to her niece Caroline her irritation almost crackles on the page: 'Your Grandmama is not *quite* well, she seldom gets through the 24 hours without some pain in her head.' Mrs Austen is a contradictory figure, though. Her nephew James records at one point that she was so ill that a short family journey could only be completed with her carried on a feather bed, but at the same time, Cassandra Leigh Austen gave birth to and raised eight children in a country parsonage, milked her own cows and enjoyed the fairly strenuous activity of cultivating potatoes. One theory for why Jane's sister destroyed so many of the author's letters after her death was that they contained too many direct or unflattering observations about their mother.

Mrs Austen 'seemed to drift more and more into a rather vaguely defined invalidism' after her children were grown up, but she still lived a long life, far outliving her husband, who died suddenly and unexpectedly at the age of seventy-five, and even surviving Jane. The author herself was frequently ill from an early age and suffered throughout her life with a chronic conjunctivitis that sometimes made it difficult for her to see well enough to read or write. She also had a bad case of 'putrid fever' when she was sent away to school at the age of seven, subsequently identified as epidemic typhus, and possibly the cause of a weakened immune system later in life. Information about her ailments is difficult to come by, however, because she kept no personal journal that we know of and her sister seems to have excised many details about her health from their letters after Jane's death.

In the last eighteen months of her life, she fell prey to a succession of infections, including an inner ear problem, shingles and childhood diseases like whooping cough, which suggest an underlying health issue that was weakening her immune system. Posthumous diagnosis has proved a popular project for biographers and doctors alike, but we have no confirmation of whether it was tuberculosis, Hodgkin's lymphoma, Addison's disease or some other illness that causes fatigue, nerve pain and immune problems. Jane herself offered a tantalising throwback to humoral theory in a letter to a friend at the start of 1817: 'I am more and more convinced that Bile is at the bottom of all I have suffered, which makes it easy to know how to treat myself,' she wrote. We do know that her declining health interfered with her ability to travel, socialise and work; at one point, she was using a pencil to write with because 'pen was become too laborious'. When she was near her end in the spring of 1817, she had to recline on 'two or three chairs' pushed together while her mother lay prostrate with some complaint or other on the sofa. This is the kind of miniature drama that so enlivens Jane's novels: I can imagine the polite utterances of *oh no, you must take the sofa, I insist* and the dark thoughts kept suppressed. Jane's niece recorded her impressions of the scene in her own memoirs:

There was only one sofa in the room – and Aunt Jane laid upon 3 chairs which she arranged for herself – I think she had a pillow, but it never looked comfortable.

Even when the sofa was vacant Jane would not use it, so as not to displace her mother as the official invalid of the house. The atmosphere becomes all the more tense when you realise that Jane was spending her time not on the sofa writing *Sanditon*, the novel she left unfinished at her death, and the entire premise of the book is the destructive power of hypochondria on a family and a community. The plot, as she had sketched it so far, centres around an attempt to turn a seaside town into a glamorous eighteenth-century watering hole and spa, with fashionable medical practitioners as one of its attractions. It ruthlessly dissects the condition of voluntary invalidism and the consumer culture that surrounds it in an extraordinary fashion. As Austen biographer Claire Tomalin puts it: 'What other fatally ill writer has embarked on a savage attack on hypochondria?'

Four months after first feeling unwell, Jane was dead at the age of forty-one. Her mother, meanwhile, lived to enjoy her sofa for another ten years, dying of old age in her late eighties. In the end, it seems as though she came to a similar accommodation with her mortality as Larkin in his final moments. 'Ah, my dear, you find me just where you left me on the sofa,' she told her grandson James Edward when he called to see her. 'I sometimes think that God Almighty must have forgotten me; but I dare say He will come for me in His own good time.'

7

We Know Too Much

I am in the belly of the machine and it is singing. The sound resonates through me, short pulses of tone and long slurs of a high-pitched wailing that haunts the edge of my hearing. My mind scrambles ineffectually against the surface of the song, wanting there to be a pattern, a motif. I count notes and try to hold frequencies in my head for comparison, but to no avail. The song slides through me and I cannot hold on to it.

A voice cuts in, irritable and crackly with static. 'Can you hold your feet still? We can see your socks moving on the monitor.' The transporting spell of the song is broken and I can feel my own body again, laid out face down on a hard plastic stretcher. The moulded ridges jut into my ribs, bruising. The fibres of my face mask tickle my nose. My arms, stretched over my head and pulled taut, tremble with the effort it takes to keep still. I am a supplicant, prostrate before the machine, begging it for knowledge.

I am inside a camera, a robot, a supercomputer, a room-sized magnet. I am made of flesh and bone and gristle and guts and hair, and I have been slotted inside to be transformed, for fractions of seconds at a time, into glass. The machine will look through me. Whatever lies beneath will be exposed to its uncaring view. The images will be beamed back to a screen in another room, where a person I'll never meet will stare at this intensely private version of me, manipulating, rotating and interpreting my body from within.

For the duration of the song, my existence has multiplied. I am a lump of meat on a slab and I am an invisible pulse of data, flowing down cables and through the atmosphere. I hover in between, aware of everything but knowing nothing. The very air of this room is alive with the tiny glass shards of me. They are dancing and twinkling invisibly under the fluorescent lights.

I am inside the machine because there is something wrong with me that nobody can see.

The first time it happened, I was on the bus. It was raining and the breath from all of us inside had steamed up the windows so that we were travelling in a blurry bubble with no connection to the outside world. I had been half listening to half of somebody else's phone call, idly imagining the sympathetic replies to their detailed descriptions of a colleague's many transgressions, when I suddenly went deaf.

No; not deaf. I could still hear the thrum of my own heart in my ears, the accelerating whoosh of my blood as my fear pumped faster and faster. A high-pitched whine emerged too, a mosquito in surround sound. That's when I stopped being able to see.

My vision dissolved into a prismatic sphere of light, a sparkling circle of refracted rays that pushed out everything else. I blinked to clear it. It was still there, stronger and brighter. I shook my head, turned towards the window, stared up into the strip lighting overhead, but there was no change. It was like looking at a disco ball turned inside out. My mouth tasted dry and rusty, my tongue sharp with fear. I felt no pain but every inch of me prickled with the awareness that something had misfired inside me. I was broken. I was certain.

I stumbled off the bus at the next stop, using the barely apparent yellow of the handrails to bounce down the aisle and out onto the pavement. My glowing, throbbing vision became even more brilliant in the full daylight. I didn't realise that I was crying, leaning against the bus shelter to stay upright, until a woman in a suit stopped to give me a bottle of water and a packet of tissues. 'I think you need this, love. Small sips,' she said as she was sucked back into the flow of commuters marching away down the hill.

I slid down to sit on the wet pavement and took a long glug of water. The edges of my glittering world softened a little and some of the grey sky seeped back into my vision. A few minutes and some more gulps later, I could hear the traffic splashing past and feel how wet my coat was from sitting on the ground. A clear patch was growing in my eyes, a tunnel through the writhing ring of light. I got to my feet and walked the rest of the way to work, waiting for a pain to set in that didn't come.

It happened three more times that week, the sudden loss of hearing and sight. There was no pattern to it, nor was I stressed or under strain when it came; on one occasion I was woken up from sleep by the whining noise and opened my eyes to see nothing but stars. Once it came on during a meeting and I just carried on nodding and smiling as if I could hear what was being said to me or see who was saying it. Nobody noticed a thing.

The fear of the attacks was far worse than the attacks themselves. Hours spent searching combinations of keywords like 'sudden deafness + sparkly eyes' online did nothing but add a sick note of anxiety to the cacophony of alarms constantly ringing in my head. Too uncertain of what was happening, if anything really was, to seek medical help, I attempted to soothe myself with information I found on the internet. I tried to become an expert in something that I was barely sure existed, these transient sensations of being trapped inside my own body, unable to see or hear. On the basis of a few searches, I did eliminate some possibilities: the lack of escalation after my symptoms began made me fairly confident that I wasn't having a stroke, a panic attack or an aneurysm. I wasn't losing consciousness, experiencing any pain, throwing up or remaining debilitated for more than a quarter of an hour. I had no localised symptoms to point to, such as numbness or tingling in any one limb. But every time I ruled out another possibility the internet threw up as a likely cause of my symptoms, my tension heightened. I was adrift in the unknown, being pulled by an inexorable current towards the rocks of some rare, elusive and probably fatal disease.

The fifth time, I came very close to falling down the stairs at my office building because I couldn't see where the top step was. Before the jolt of terror could subside, I seized the brief sense of certainty that there must really be something detectable causing these attacks and used it as a sign that I should call a doctor. At the late evening appointment, chosen so that I would not have to tell anybody at work that I might be sick, a bored-looking locum listened to my halting account of the problem. She asked me general questions about diet, exercise, stress. Her screen was angled away from me, but I could see the reflection in the dark window behind her; she was following a script, inputting my responses and then asking whatever query the software suggested next. It quickly became clear that I didn't fit into any of the pathways laid out within the programme, because it kept taking us around in circles, suggesting the same questions in the hope of different responses. I left with no answers and a full diary of medical tests and explorations, the attendance of which came with an added layer of stress, since I couldn't bear to explain to my roommates or colleagues what was going on: I crept around London's hospitals like a spy on a secret mission, using as few of the paid sick days I was lucky to have as possible.

I became a shadow person who existed only to be pricked, scanned and quantified, a minuscule data point in the NHS's vast diagnostic machine. I saw a nutritionist, a neurologist, a urologist, a cardiologist, a psychiatrist and an endocrinologist. Each appointment opened the same way: with the specialist's pen poised over a blank sheet of paper, awaiting my story. There were no computer screens between us now, but I still felt like I was trapped in a maze not of my making. What they said depended upon what I said, and the pressure gave me a paralysing sort of performance anxiety, as if someone else could be doing a better job of describing my own sensations. Even though these appointments were completely free – and I was aware of the extraordinary privilege I had in being able to access expert healthcare like this without having to consider the finances of it all – I went into each one so nervous I could barely speak. I felt both pulled towards those rooms and pushed away from them. I wanted to quell my constant fear by finding out what was wrong with me and I believed that these experts were the ones to do it, but I also wished I had a life that didn't involve this constant cycle of assessment and uncertainty.

As no cause of the episodes emerged, the tests became more detailed, intensive and specialised. I collected all of my urine for forty-eight hours in a giant vat so heavy that I had to strap it to the front of my bicycle and wheel it along the pavement so that I could drop it off awkwardly at the clinic reception. I wore a heart monitor for a week that gave me an angry red rash where it made contact with my skin. I spent a day and a night hooked up to a portable blood pressure machine that gripped my arm, vice-like, every thirty minutes. I was shut inside a small shower cubicle and told to hold my breath while the efficiency of my lungs was measured. Ultrasound probes were run over my kidneys, my liver, my heart.

I continued to see the sparkly vision a few times a week, except now I knew that it was called an 'aura'. Doctors drew diagrams of my body for me on scrap paper, their scribbled arrows illustrating theories about why I might be having these sudden periods of involuntarily depressed brain activity. Tumours on my kidneys, lungs and brain were hypothesised, which then melted into air when they did not show up on any of the scans. My symptoms weren't progressing, but neither were they going away. I was stuck in limbo, with every appointment spawning at least three others.

None of my tests had showed anything unusual. Which is how I ended up inside an MRI machine for ninety minutes, my veins throbbing with an injected contrast material, waiting to see if something would finally be revealed. Even while lying motionless I was oscillating constantly between two contradictory yet desperate hopes: I really wanted the scan to find something, so that I would finally have a name to put to my nameless symptoms, and I was terrified that the scan would deliver the devastating news that I had some life-altering illness. And even as I bounced between these two different desires, something else niggled at me. Could I even be satisfied with the results? Or would my hypochondriacal impulses always convince me that there was something else lurking, unseen, just out of reach?

Since hypochondria was uncoupled from its medieval association with the hypochondrium region of the upper abdomen, it has existed increasingly only as a concept, rather than a physical, visible entity. But now, it isn't even that. The last great transition of hypochondria has made it disappear: no longer can a patient walk out of a consulting room with that diagnosis newly attached to their records and their psyche. The *DSM-5* prefers 'illness anxiety disorder' and 'somatic symptom disorder' over the 'hypochondriasis' included in previous editions, a much commented-on change from the American Psychiatric Association, which signalled a more general international appetite to dispense with a term that was felt to be vague, old-fashioned, clinically unhelpful and mired in stigma. When speaking generally of an excessive preoccupation with illness, the vast majority of physicians and therapists will now speak of 'health anxiety' rather than hypochondria, preferring not to touch the old word for fear the patient will feel judged or belittled as a malingerer. This is confirmed in the latest version of the World Health Organization's International Classification of Diseases, published in 2022, which made 'health anxiety disorder' an interchangeable term for hypochondriasis, which was in turn subsumed under obsessive compulsive disorder.

In keeping with the scattered, disputed definitions of hypochondria in the past, there is not much settled agreement on what 'health anxiety' even is, despite its frequent and widespread use. Some experts use the two terms interchangeably, as a like-for-like replacement, while others see them as overlapping but distinct phenomena. If health anxiety is just any worry about anything to do with health, then some degree of it can be 'considered normal', as one researcher puts it – it is natural to feel slightly concerned about an oncoming cold if you feel a tickle in the throat, say. This kind of worry can usually be soothed once the physical symptoms are relieved; there is no anxiety attached to the overarching concept of illness, so a few painkillers and a good night's rest will sort it out. It is only when the concern has 'exceeded the normal range' that this natural health anxiety becomes hypochondria. Then the preoccupation is with finding the underlying cause of the symptoms, and relieving the symptoms themselves will do nothing to alleviate the anxiety. This obsessive desire for knowledge manifests as a symptom of its own. Precisely where this boundary between normal and abnormal lies is not clear, though. Exactly what level of anxiety causes this profound shift in mindset has yet to be determined.

This is not through lack of attempts, though. Questionnaires are a long-standing tool in psychology as a way of extracting consistent information from patients, as they enable self-reporting while keeping the responses structured around key questions. Each answer can be weighted and scored, so that when totalled the results place the participant somewhere on a numerical scale that represents the severity of their condition. The scores cannot be treated as objective data, though, since they reveal what the patient *thinks* is happening rather than anything else. One interesting study on the effectiveness of questionnaires for testing memory loss found that people consistently think that their memory is better than it really is according to the results of other tests. Questionnaires measure belief, not actual performance. But since hypochondria and health anxiety are impossible to untangle from subjective belief about the body's sensations, this has not been a barrier to this kind of assessment. For half a century now, researchers have been devising questionnaires aimed at discovering the degree of health anxiety a patient is experiencing. Issy Pilowsky's Whiteley Index (WI) first appeared in 1967, and included questions like 'Do you often worry about the possibility that you have got a serious illness?' and 'Do you think that you worry about your health more than most people?' It enquires into three different dimensions of anxiety about health: fear of disease; preoccupation with somatic, or unexplained, symptoms; and disease conviction – the belief that a particular disease has already been contracted, despite evidence to the contrary. The WI has been supplemented with further questions since, resulting in the development of the Illness Behaviour Questionnaire in the 1970s, the Illness Attitude Scale in the 1980s, and most recently the Hypochondriasis Yale-Brown Obsessive-Compulsive Scale, but the original version in a truncated six-question form is still found to be useful as an opening assessment. As imprecise and subjective as this kind of measurement is, it is still the best option we have for trying to turn such a personal, internal condition into external data that clinicians can use.

Changing the terminology and using questionnaires don't relieve the anxiety about not being believed, though. This is so intrinsic to hypochondria and health anxiety that the WI includes it as one of the possible indicators: 'Do you get the feeling that people are not taking your illness seriously enough?', it asks. Anxiety as a symptom of anxiety. Every conversation I have had with a hypochondriac while writing this book has been peppered with stories about being dismissed, ignored and sent away when seeking help. I have spoken with people now living with long-term, life-altering diagnoses of conditions like multiple sclerosis and Parkinson's disease who, when they initially presented their symptoms to doctors, were told – because of their previous anxiety – to stop inventing problems where

there were none. I think constantly about a story the writer
Leslie Jamison tells in her book *The Recovering*, when, after
living in South America, she returns home to the US convinced
that she has a botfly larva growing inside her ankle. After much
dismissal by experts of her concerns, a dermatologist eventually
confirms Jamison's supposedly outlandish theories in the most
disgustingly visceral way: by pulling the creature out of her
body with tweezers. And yet she is barely comforted at all by
this resolution, or by being proved right against the odds. She
is immediately sunk into terror that there is another botfly in
there, right underneath where the first one was. The negative
reinforcement and shame are so powerful.

This official transition from 'hypochondria' to 'health
anxiety' suggests that there has been a modernisation of the
condition, a great advance in understanding, but a change
in vocabulary cannot shift the residue of centuries of deeply
rooted ideas about what is real and what is not, and what is
deserving of medical attention. Another increasingly used term
for the hypochondriac or health-anxious segment of society is
the 'worried well'. This phrase is usually deployed by health
policymakers and clinicians in a negative context; the idea that
these people are worrying over nothing is built into this combination of words. It has no official definition but is normally
applied in situations where a doctor cannot discern any physiological cause for the symptoms the patient describes – this may
be because of a complex or early-onset condition that requires
more sensitive tests, or it may be because of hypochondria.
The worried well are a problem to policymakers because they
overuse medical services trying to get answers about their
elusive conditions. This perception can in turn result in poorer
medical outcomes. 'The more popular the term becomes, the
easier it is for doctors who cannot quickly identify physical

signs of disease to label the patient as "the worried well",' a distinguished retired British GP wrote in 2020. He argued that making value judgements about who is more worthy of medical treatment risks reinstating the prejudices of decades past about the 'deserving and undeserving poor' and ultimately undermines patients' trust in their doctors.

And there is also the risk that the fear of being made to feel frivolous or wasteful for taking up resources is preventing people from seeking help. By the time I was a few years past my cancer all-clear, I had internalised this thought pattern so much that I was also avoiding the doctor for standard routine monitoring procedures like smear tests and eschewing dental appointments completely for fear of wasting experts' valuable time. To be clear: no medical professional had ever actually described me as one of the 'worried well'; my medical history usually gives me an aura of plausibility as a patient that I may or may not deserve. But a combination of stories from friends about how their urgent questions about symptoms and medication side effects – especially women concerned about the effects various contraceptive drugs and devices were having on their bodies – had been summarily dismissed, and my personality's inherent need to not be a bother to anyone had given me a highly strung fear of being accused of misusing medical resources.

Hypochondria puts doctors in a very difficult situation. Patients come seeking reassurance and definitive answers to questions that likely have none. Their every expression can make the situation worse: be too brisk, and the patient may feel dismissed or belittled; be too solicitous and risk encouraging an unhealthy pattern of behaviour. Any suggestion that what the patient believes to be their illness is not real can result in turning them off from even responsible maintenance of their health.

Research suggests that sending a hypochondriac for further, unjustified tests just to allay their fears in fact only heightens their anxiety. Other than prescribing directly for health anxiety, one of the few accepted strategies for dealing with it can be so-called benign remedies – recommending things like vitamins, heating pads, or exercises that can do no harm even if what they are treating does not exist, while making the patient feel like their doctor takes them seriously and is trying to help.

By my mid-twenties, I had started applying this anxiety about being branded a time-waster to other kinds of emergencies too. One Saturday night, other tenants higher up in the block of flats where I lived started setting fire to pieces of furniture and throwing them off the balcony – my flatmate and I watched, horrified, as flaming chairs fell past our windows and hit the ground in an explosion of sparks. The hallway was smoky, too. We agonised about whether to call the fire service; nothing structural was actually *on fire*, after all, and I was paranoid that we would be told off for wasting the time of an overstretched emergency service. Finally, we settled on calling the non-emergency police number, so that they at least had the incident on record. A bored-sounding operator took down the details, and we returned to watching television, ignoring the sparks and the smoke streaking the night sky outside. About five minutes later, two fire engines roared up to the building, all sirens blazing, and suited-up officers began checking each floor for problems. When they were finished and the pyromaniacs on the floor above had been duly dealt with, the captain came to speak to us. He was very gentle, but he made it clear that by *not* calling the emergency number immediately, we had delayed the response by what could have been crucial minutes if one of the flaming chairs had hit the building or someone walking below, for instance. Ever since, I have felt trapped between the two possible courses of action: should I treat everything as a potential emergency, or nothing? Gripped by this dilemma, it is little wonder that people live in a frustrated state of hyper-alertness with their health.

The modern world continually provides reminders that we ought to be monitoring our health, whether that comes from charity awareness campaigns, public information about positive lifestyle changes or our own digital devices, which are now capable of automatically chiding us when we don't take enough steps every hour or we drink too little water. So much of modern life is now quantified, providing data points with which amateur clinicians like me can diagnose themselves. Steps are tracked, sleep is logged, calories are counted. The smartphones that are never far from our hands aid and abet us in this great collection of data. Thumbing through the preinstalled apps on a new phone, it's too easy to pause over the one labelled 'Health'. I remember opening it for the first time and feeling startled to see a line representing my heartbeat wriggling across the screen and a graph beneath showing how many steps I had taken so far that day. Without my even being aware of it, I was being flattened into numbers and trends. Although a fitness tracker is no replacement for proper medical monitoring, there is an extent to which this kind of data helps to democratise health – allowing people to see information about their bodies without having to enter an intimidating, and often expensive, medical institution. Having more good information can be a useful tool when managing health anxiety, too. After some CBT sessions to help with insomnia, I was advised to wear a tracker on my wrist while I slept and check how many hours of slumber it had recorded every night. The idea was that this would prevent me spiralling into extremes: rather than telling myself 'I didn't sleep at all', I could see that I'd got four and a half hours last night, which, while not ideal, is also not nothing. As with so many elements of hypochondria, though, the line between helpful inquiry and unhealthy obsession is easy to cross. I eventually had to retire my tracker after it began to feed rather than soothe my anxiety. Day after day of failing to turn green the red circles in the app representing my lack of deep sleep and healthy movement made me feel worse about my state of health, not better.

The idea that we should be able to diagnose disease before we feel its effects is a new one – until the last few decades, a lack of symptoms was considered to be a good indication of a lack of illness. One of the miracles of modern medicine is that disease can now be detected at the cellular level, long before it develops into a fever that weakens or a mass that can be palpated. Hypochondria has also changed to incorporate this new phenomenon; the potential for anxiety has become so much greater now that it is legitimately possible to have a verifiable condition without yet exhibiting any symptoms. Every queasy feeling or odd inner lurch could be the first sign of some deeper malfunction, and in some cases doctors have even begun to tell patients to be alert for such early warning signs. As testing methods have improved and public education about early warning signs has expanded, medicine has gradually shifted from being reactive to being preventative.

Public health is the term used for the organised, large-scale measures taken to ensure that a population is protected against threats to its health. Vaccination programmes are one of the most visible ways that this manifests in day-to-day life, but health education and 'invisible' interventions like adding fluoride to the water supply are part of it too. The shift from an individual to a collective understanding of what it means to be healthy was brought about by two principal factors – what is known as 'the great sanitary awakening' of the mid-nineteenth century when links were first made between the spread of disease and personal (and spiritual) cleanliness, and the rise of preventative medicine. Dirt and filth were identified as both a cause of sickness and a way in which it was spread, from which ideas of sanitation and hygiene for the public good grew. The way we think about public health today – as part of the social contract and our responsibility to each other – has its origins in this shift during the nineteenth century. We monitor sanitary conditions and levels of disease on a population level so as to have the best possible chance of keeping the most people alive for the longest time. The increased focus on public health has overwhelmingly improved quality of life and life expectancy, and there is plenty of evidence showing that public monitoring and advance screening programmes reduce the overall number of fatalities from what are now avoidable conditions. It's also big business: in the US alone, the preventative healthcare and services market is predicted to be worth $432.4 billion by 2024. Reassurance is always available to those who are willing to pay for it. In a scene from the reality television series *The Kardashians*, multi-millionaire matriarch Kris Jenner visits a clinic that offers elective full-body scans that claim to be able to pick up on health problems before a patient has any reason to go to their normal physician. 'What we sell here is peace of mind,' the attendant tells Jenner as she arrives. I wonder if the opposite is actually true.

Once again, hypochondria is the ghost at the feast, casting doubt upon medicine's onward march. For someone disposed towards health anxiety, the constant pressure to participate in public health programmes can be a huge mental burden – an omnipresent reminder that at every moment there might be something wrong with you. Regular invitations to attend mammograms and blood tests tear jagged holes in the fragile carapace of 'health' that a sufferer has painstakingly built up. They cause unanswerable questions to bounce around the mind. Why would they ask me to do this test if there wasn't a chance that it could find something bad?

And it is no longer just hypochondriacs who are aware of this effect. Medical authorities in the US and the UK are now beginning to closely examine and even scale back on mass screening programmes for conditions like breast and prostate cancers, as recognition of the mental and physical harms such tests can cause grows. Once thought to be a universal positive if they catch disease early, researchers are now beginning to think that the negative consequences (extra radiation from scans, the mental health toll of waiting for results, the unnecessary surgeries that happen when small, harmless masses are detected) might outweigh the population-level benefits. The presence of the profit motive once again makes everything more complicated, because in a market-driven healthcare system such as the one in the US, there is a clear commercial incentive for providers to convince patients that they need elective scans and tests 'just in case', and even some evidence to suggest that such ready access to diagnostics creates health anxiety in people who had never previously experienced it. The hypochondriac with comprehensive health insurance is the holy grail patient. It's an impossible calculus, and one that the hypochondriac attempts every single day: which risk is worse? Knowing, or not knowing?

'Don't google your cancer,' the oncology nurse said to me as she swabbed my arm with alcohol for the first of many blood tests that would determine exactly how toxic my treatment could be without killing me. There was a pause while she picked up new equipment from the tray beside us, the familiar rattle of metal against metal loud in the silent room. As she turned back to me and the needle went in, she continued. 'But if you really, really have to look online, please only look at the sites that I've printed out for you.' She did not elaborate on what might happen if I broke these rules; it was clear that she thought the consequences were so obvious and dire that they didn't need explanation. When I left the clinic that day, I took with me this list of approved resources, which included the NHS website, a patient's guide published by a cancer charity, a couple of online medical dictionaries and some academic publishers where I could access relevant scientific papers. The web addresses were long and nonsensical, strings of meaningless letters and numbers spilling across the page; nobody was yet used to the idea that such things needed to be easily shareable. I handed this document over to my parents, where it was pinned on the cork noticeboard in the kitchen with all of the other boring but important information related to my new status as a cancer patient.

This was in 2006. I wouldn't own a smartphone for another three years. I'd never even seen one. I didn't have a portable device that could connect to the internet at all. All of my online existence occurred either via the family desktop computer in the study downstairs, or in the communal computer room at school. I associated these bulky, cream plastic boxes almost exclusively with homework or occasionally messaging my friends if we happened to be online at the same time. Freeform research on any topic was done in a library. My brain still operated on the basis that if I wanted to know something, I had to wait until I was next in front of a screen, which might not be until the next day. The instant gratification loop I inhabit today, where my every query can be satisfied within seconds by a device that hardly ever leaves my hand, did not yet exist.

The peculiar thing to me now is that I never did google my cancer. I think my father made use of that list of recommended websites to answer some of his own questions about survival rates and environmental causes, but I asked him not to tell me about what he found out. I had an oddly sponge-like memory as a teenager – a faculty that has long since ebbed away with age – and I used to remember everything that my doctors and nurses said to me, verbatim. When I went to bed after a long day at the hospital I would replay everything that had been said, filtering out all words that seemed comforting or positive and filing them away carefully in my head. I was satisfied with the numbers and probabilities that the consultant threw out in our meetings, so I never felt the urge to look for alternatives. If he said that ninety-five per cent of people who were diagnosed with this kind of cancer at my age were cured by the first round of chemotherapy, then that was all I needed to know.

My trust was broken when that treatment did not work. I was in the unlucky five per cent, the doctor said, laying out his plans for a more aggressive course of chemotherapy that required overnight stays in the hospital and a subsequent stem cell transplant. A year had passed; I was no longer a schoolgirl but a university student, and now I had my own laptop. I was free to search 'cancer death rates age 18' as much as I liked, and click, and click, and click, until I had to close the lid of the computer to stop the tears falling into the keyboard. I didn't blame my doctor for the cancer's re-emergence – my research revealed to me that he had been correct in laying out the probabilities – but I no longer felt satisfied in the role of passive patient who is only given as much information as those in charge judge that she can handle. I had so little control over the rest of my life, unable to say from one week to the next what I would be capable of doing, that seeking out knowledge about what was going on in my body felt like a small measure of resistance against the circumstances that had blanked out my entire future.

When I was given the all-clear and discharged from further follow-up appointments, this habit remained of opening up a new search engine window whenever I felt like something was a bit off. I did it constantly, often spending nights under the covers with my phone screen lighting up my face as I read academic papers about nerve degeneration or surfed my way through obscure forums where people shared pictures of their rashes for others to diagnose. Having starved myself of this glut of material before, I gorged on it as much as possible. The accident of timing and technological progress meant that I experienced patienthood both ways: without the internet and then with it, and I think the sudden conversion from one state to the other made me an addict.

The internet became a big part of the rituals that I built around my health anxieties, a way in which I convinced myself that I was handling it 'properly'. I was raised by scientists and taught always to trust evidence over assertion. Never mind the fact that I always eventually logged off feeling far worse than when I started, because my every search pulled up a spiralling string of suggestions that accelerated in severity as I eliminated the most common explanations. If hypochondria is a performance, then I needed material. I was oddly dispassionate and calculating about this, even as the panic sang loudly in my ears. I had to have a frame of reference to know how afraid I should be. I needed to accumulate the right language so that if I ever spoke to a medical professional about my current problem, I would be able to make them understand what was happening. I had spent three years studying for a university degree that made it very clear that it was not possible to read too many books. Later I worked as a journalist and an editor, relentlessly asking the question 'what's your source for this?' I absorbed into my identity the lie that this health 'research' was similarly legitimate. I was just being responsible. How could trying to be well informed be a bad thing?

The contradictory role of information in the perception of health is a big part of hypochondria as we know it today. On the one hand, knowing more about what goes on inside our bodies – transforming them from opaque meat sacks into transparent, comprehensible glass figures – seems like an unequivocally positive development. If progress happens over time, surely it is because we know more than we did before. But there is a darker and more dangerous side to all this knowledge: the idea that learning *about* a particular illness can make you believe that you *have* said illness. If I didn't know cancer existed, would I fear that I had it? Does my intimate knowledge of the way tumours are detected and excised make me more prone to believing they are there? The way that hypochondriacal fears have kept pace with technology throughout history would suggest 'no' for the first question and 'yes' for the second question: I can only worry about what I already know is possibly lurking in my body. I need to understand a disease before I can be scared of it. And if that is the case, then perhaps ignorance is bliss when it comes to health.

Hypochondriacs are hypervigilant about potential bodily malfunction, but it is true that we also live with an ear perpetually cocked for information about some new disease that might explain everything that feels wrong inside. We are voracious consumers of stories about health. Anything will do: an anecdote from a colleague about a sister-in-law who had a stroke after thinking that her eyes were just strained from too much computer work; an article in the newspaper about a newly discovered virus; a conversation overheard on the bus about mild chest pains that resulted in emergency open-heart surgery. Being confronted with the story of an illness, in any form, can be enough to plant the seed that blooms into that fatal question: do I have it?

Part of this can be attributed to our perpetual desire to find meaning in apparently meaningless incidents, as well as a natural inclination to give more weight to negative information than positive. The brain instinctively latches on to anything that might provide that yearned-for explanation that unites the aching eyes, the mild vertigo and the sore knee. Accepting that the body is a wildly complicated and mysterious entity composed of many overlapping systems that can misfire at any moment for no discernible reason and without seeking any permission from the consciousness that inhabits it is far less satisfying than believing in a grand unified theory that governs it all. And there's nothing we can do about that, really. As John Green, author of multiple novels about the quotidian horror and joy of inhabiting a less than perfect body and mind, once put it: 'I don't believe we have a choice when it comes to whether we endow the world with meaning. We are all little fairies, sprinkling meaning dust everywhere we go.'

Learning about a particular condition, then, can seem like a way of providing a structure upon which all the disparate elements can hang. That same suggestibility that makes sleight-of-hand magic tricks work on me every single time is present here too. *I do have a sore wrist a lot of the time*, I'm thinking while someone is telling me about their cousin's juvenile arthritis diagnosis. Likewise, I had never been worried that I had polycystic ovarian syndrome until a friend mentioned that she had been diagnosed with it. Then I fell down an internet rabbit hole of gruesome pictures of cysts that resulted in me getting two ultrasounds, one internal and one external, to rule it out as an explanation for my intermittently present fatigue, hair loss and skin issues. It's a way of mitigating the isolation of living with the unknown: *perhaps I am just like her,* is what I am really wondering. Once more, a combination of my history with cancer and my good fortune to live in a less overstretched healthcare region at a time when the NHS was under less intense pressure than it is now acted like a magic key to unlock the mysteries of the healthcare system: this was all done promptly and for free, a blessing, albeit a slightly mixed one, for the hypochondriac.

And it is not just laypeople who are prone to this. There is a much-documented effect among medical students known col-loquially as 'medical student syndrome', where those learning about diseases are prone to developing the incapacitating belief that they have contracted said diseases. It is sometimes called 'intern's syndrome' or 'second year syndrome', in reference to the stage of training at which this hypochondriacal phenome-non typically surfaces. The assumption is that these trainees, who of course have to digest an enormous quantity and variety of information about different diseases and ailments in order to obtain their qualifications, at a certain point will succumb to the suggestion that they are experiencing them too. The stressful and competitive nature of medical study is also considered to be a factor, conjuring up an image of an overworked and over-tired student with a brain stuffed full of horrifying medical facts cracking under the pressure and unconsciously seeking a legitimate way of taking a break – that is, being mortally ill.

The anecdotal presence of this condition around the world is sufficiently high that it has even been included on the syllabus for psychology studies at multiple institutions. Unsurprisingly, doctors and researchers are quite interested in this cognitive feedback loop that seems to be going on within their ranks, so there have been a few attempts to reproduce its effects in a more rigorous environment. There is an attractive circularity about this syndrome that invites inquiry: what if 'physician, heal thyself' is a more literal injunction than we realise? Multiple studies from the last decade, however, have failed to find any evidence that medical students are more inclined towards hypochondria than the average population. The persistence of this myth, though, can do harm in and of itself if it discourages medical students from seeking treatment for their ailments from fear that they will be dismissed as merely suffering from this syndrome. Even the suggestion that such a condition might exist is enough to have a lasting impact on the way the medical practitioners of the future view the validity of their own health concerns, and by extension, those of their patients. The link between too much knowledge of health problems and the problems themselves is embedded in the atmosphere of medical education.

The intensely suggestive power of medical knowledge is an issue that long predates the internet, although our perpetually online lives today make it feel more present and urgent. In the novel *Three Men in a Boat*, first published in 1889, Jerome K. Jerome provides the perfect case study of this page-to-plague effect. The book begins with the narrator (also called Jerome) spending an evening at his lodgings in London with two friends and his dog. The trio of young men are 'feeling seedy' and 'getting quite nervous about it' as they each describe their maladies to an audience of the other two. Harris experiences great fits of giddiness and disorientation, and George quickly says that he has precisely the same symptoms and sensations, although it is later confided to the reader that he is the real hypochondriac of the bunch: 'George *fancies* he is ill; but there's never anything really the matter with him, you know.' Jerome, meanwhile, is struggling with his liver: the classical hypochondriac concern. He has diagnosed this problem for himself after reading a circular that described all of the symptoms of an out-of-order liver. 'It is a most extraordinary thing, but I never read a patent medicine advertisement without being impelled to the conclusion that I am suffering from the particular disease therein dealt with in its most virulent form,' he reflects. 'The diagnosis seems in every case to correspond exactly with all the sensations that I have ever felt.' He also recalls a previous occasion when he took himself to the reading room at the British Museum to read up on the symptoms of some long-forgotten malady. The book he ends up consulting is a medical dictionary, and on his way to finding the entry he was seeking, he finds himself distracted by all the other diseases itemised within. He reads them all and finds that he is sickening for everything; he has been coming down with this alphabetical cocktail of ailments for months, in fact. The book condemns him to the state of helpless invalid. 'I had walked into that reading-room a happy, healthy man. I crawled out a decrepit wreck.'

Over a hundred years later, the writer John O'Connell had a very similar experience to Jerome. In 2005's *I Told You I Was Ill*, he writes about the childhood origins of his hypochondria. It partly stemmed from watching documentaries on television: an episode of the long-running BBC science series *Horizon* which included footage from inside a patient suffering from severe heart disease gave him, at eleven years old, a mortal fear of cholesterol that prevented him from taking a single bite of the vanilla millefeuille slice his mother bought as a regular Saturday treat. I had a similar experience myself at around the same age; while my family was on holiday in Germany we ate at a restaurant that had on its menu a dessert named *Tod durch Schokolade*, or 'death by chocolate'. I shared a portion with my father, and then stared wide-eyed and rigid with fright at the ceiling all night waiting for the reaper to come for me. The cake had been rich and dark and covered in cream, and according to my naive logic the adults who made it wouldn't name it as a cause of death unless they had good reason. Needless to say, I did not die as a consequence of the cake, and the following morning my parents explained the concepts of 'black humour' and 'hyperbole' to me.

While O'Connell is in the grip of his self-imposed low-cholesterol diet, he receives a book as a Christmas present: *The Pears Encyclopaedia of Child Health*. This gift, given to encourage his nascent interest in medicine so that he might one day follow in the footsteps of a doctor grandfather, changes everything. 'From this moment on, hypochondria gatecrashes my life,' he explains. 'Thousands of tiny health-related worries appear out of nowhere and assume elephantine proportions.' Every single ordinary thing he does in the day now carries the potential to make him seriously ill. He can't drink coffee (risk of heart attack), stroke the family cat (might get toxoplasmosis) or eat white bread (the lack of fibre might cause his rectum to prolapse, the worst thing that could possibly happen to him). In the *Encyclopaedia*, he has an authoritative guide to everything that could go wrong with his body. His every fear is there, alphabetised and presented in helpfully child-friendly terms. The dangers of high cholesterol, however, are omitted – no doubt because it is not considered a major factor for the book's focus of child health. O'Connell is so worried about this oversight that he writes to the authors to correct them. They never reply to his letter.

*

This negative power of suggestion has a name: the nocebo reaction. It is often described as the negative counterpart or 'evil twin' of the placebo effect. It was first identified and named by Dr Walter Kennedy in 1961, who was looking specifically at the impact of negative expectation on the likelihood of an unpleasant response to a medication. Whereas a placebo can cause a patient to experience the positive benefits of a drug when they are not actually consuming it, a nocebo does the opposite. If given a harmless sugar pill and told that it is a drug with potentially harmful side effects, the patient may experience those symptoms, despite never having ingested the substance that causes them. Kennedy coined the term from a Latin verb, *nocero*, meaning 'to harm', to contrast with *placeo*, 'to please', the root of the word 'placebo'.

Subsequent studies have found plenty of evidence for the nocebo response. One early trial from 1968 on patients with breathing issues like asthma or emphysema found that if these sufferers were exposed to a gas made from nebulising a harmless saline solution but told that they were inhaling an allergen or irritant, almost half of them would experience coughing, wheezing and other responses associated with a genuine reaction. Further to this, twelve of the forty participants in the study developed full-blown bronchospasm attacks, which were then treated successfully with the same nebulised saline solution that had caused the problem in the first place – the only difference being that this time they were told they were receiving Isuprel, a drug that was commonly used at the time for treating asthma.

Meanwhile, none of the healthy people in the control group reacted at all. The negative expectations of those with pre-existing conditions that caused breathing difficulties, in other words, caused them to experience symptoms that were consistent with what they were told, rather than what their body actually ingested. I witnessed this for myself, after a fashion, when I worked as a stage manager for theatre productions at school. We had a very basic smoke machine that pumped out steam infused with a small amount of non-toxic glycerin solution to give it a foggy colour and texture. It was entirely possible to breathe this in without even noticing the change in air quality, as I found while operating it backstage – it looked like smoke but it was really just coloured vapour, similar to what might be given off by a boiling kettle. I knew this, of course, because I had prepared the solution and poured it into the machine. The audience, however, used to react as if it was the intense smoke that it appeared to be. Night after night, I used to watch in bewilderment as the vapour would drift slowly out from the stage into the hall and, row by row, audience members would start to cough furiously. They took their cue from the actors, who were of course pretending that the smoke was real, and the fact that it *looked* like real smoke, ignoring the sensation of what their bodies were really inhaling.

A recent review of randomised trials related to the side effects of Covid vaccinations found a very similar effect. All participants were carefully informed about all the potentially adverse effects, but were not told whether they were receiving the actual vaccine or a harmless placebo. The negative side effects were categorised into two groups: systemic events, such as headaches or fatigue, and local ones, such as temporary inflammation or aching at the injection site. A startlingly high seventy-six per cent of systemic side effects experienced after a first dose could be attributed to the nocebo effect, while by contrast just 24.3 per cent of local issues were prompted by the dummy vaccine. The researchers hypothesised that this is because it is much easier for patients to misattribute generalised or unexplained weariness and pain to a recent vaccine, whereas an ache in the specific area of the arm that the needle penetrated is harder to talk yourself into. Anxiety and stress are also known to cause systemic symptoms like headache and fatigue, meaning that the response thought to be associated with receiving the vaccine could well just be occurring as a result of worrying about the vaccine.

The same effect has been detected with diseases, not just treatments. Most anxiety disorders share common symptoms with heart disease, such as breathlessness, palpitations, chest pains and nausea. A 2016 Norwegian study tested the hypothesis that there is a link between health anxiety specifically and a greater risk of heart disease, the idea being that if you worry about contracting it, you are more likely to contract it. Using the WI to identify over 7,000 patients with high levels of health anxiety, researchers then explored their subsequent medical records and compared incidents of heart disease to the population baseline. The results showed that those with health anxiety were seventy-three per cent more likely to develop heart disease over a period of ten years – a figure that is so eye-catchingly high that it even received some attention in the mainstream, non-medical media upon publication. In an attempt to find an explanation for this data other than the power of fear and negative expectation, the researchers examined the lifestyles of their health anxiety cohort to see if there was a high rate of other heart disease co-morbidities. Overall, compared with those without health anxiety, this group reported doing fewer hours of physical activity and a higher rate of smoking, but a lower rate of alcohol consumption. The sedentary lifestyle and the smoking are both associated with higher incidents of heart disease, and the study's authors speculated that these two habits could have been adopted specifically as a result of health anxiety. Not attempting exercise could become a habit out of 'fear of forcing or putting strain on the body', while smoking may appeal because of the sense of relaxation that nicotine provides. Alcohol, meanwhile, impairs the feeling of control over the body, and is thus less likely to appeal to those who already feel like they have little power over their symptoms.

The implications of these nocebo responses in a medical setting are tricky, especially when they inflate concerns about the adverse effects of vital vaccines and medications. For ethical reasons, patients need to be fully informed of the consequences of any substance they are receiving, but it also seems like doing so can cause people unnecessary suffering. This is still an evolving area of research, but there is some evidence that just informing people up front about the nocebo effect can help to mitigate its impact. Along with details of the drug itself and the probability of its known side effects, if patients are given information about nocebo issues and told about the difference between systemic and local effects, they are less likely to experience them than a control group that is just given the medication details. Communicating that some people experience after-effects like headaches or fatigue because of anxiety can also help, as can framing the probability of these in a positive rather than negative way – to put it simply, instead of saying 'five in a hundred people experience this', you can state that 'ninety-five in a hundred people don't experience this'. We can't eliminate the power of suggestion when it comes to our health, it seems, but we can harness it in a more optimistic direction.

The version of the nocebo effect that is specific to a particular condition or medication is closely tied to the present-day form of hypochondria, of course. Overconsumption of information about the negative consequences of symptoms and treatments is a classic presentation of the condition. It has even been incorporated into the description of 'illness anxiety disorder' in the latest edition of the *DSM-5*, which is one of the two official successor conditions to 'hypochondriasis' as defined by the American Psychiatric Association. Sufferers of this condition, we are told, 'research their suspected disease excessively (e.g., on the Internet)'. The terrifying realisation, though, is that via the nocebo effect this excessive research can be not just a symptom of hypochondria, but a foundational part of it.

Another more blurry form of the nocebo response is tied not to particular illnesses or treatments, but to any situation in which a person's negative beliefs about their wellbeing or sanity are made real merely because they believe in them. Much of the nocebo literature from the twentieth century focuses on cultures in which voodoo religions are prevalent, and cites examples where believers have died after their hair or nail clippings have been used to exert supernatural power over them, or after coming in contact with objects that they believe have been infused with the power of malevolent spirits. This effect is also associated generally with curses and prophecies: if the target of a hex does in fact suffer in the way intended, that may be because they believe in the system of power evoked. Perhaps Robert Burton truly did die of natural causes on the day that his astrologer had predicted purely because he had invested so much authority in this method of divination. A good example of this generalised anxiety can be found in the diaries of Austrian composer Joseph Haydn, who recorded in 1792 that an English clergyman had died after hearing a performance of his Symphony No. 75 in D major. This cleric had apparently dreamed the night before that a piece of music just like Haydn's slow second movement would announce his death, and upon hearing it he went home, retired to his bed and died. In a similar, albeit slightly less dramatic, fashion, someone who is mortally afraid that they will die as a consequence of a routine surgery might actually pass away in that manner, even though the operation itself goes off perfectly. In a 1961 study, researchers interviewed 600 surgical patients at Massachusetts General Hospital and isolated five who reported experiencing a profound premonition that they would die as a result of their procedure. Their subsequent medical histories were then monitored, and indeed all five did pass away during the convalescence period or shortly afterwards. Experts attributed the deaths of these patients not to physical causes, but to emotional factors that informed their belief that their life was at its end, regardless of their medical prognosis. 'Death held more appeal for these patients than did life,' one author commented, somewhat strangely. What we think and what we learn matter, more than we know. How and where we learn it matter too – and here again, the internet is key.

As an engine for perpetually presenting new material and new ways to be afraid, the internet is unbeatable. It is the most expansive and spacious playground that hypochondria has ever had. Contrary to some contemporary media narratives, hypochondria doesn't exist because of the internet. As the preceding chapters have demonstrated, it has a long heritage that far predates the raucous, oscillating song of a dial-up modem. But it has been changed and enlarged by our perpetual access to an entire universe of information. It has fundamentally shifted the relationship between patient and doctor. There used to be a substantial difference between the level of medical knowledge accessible to the average layperson and that held by someone with medical training and degrees; now with a few taps I can have the same textbooks and scientific papers in front of me that medical students are perusing. Perhaps more importantly, I can also access a wealth of less regulated material, ranging from well-meaning websites to deliberate disinformation, all targeted at my fears about my health. A doctor nearing retirement once summed this up for me: 'Patients used to come in to ask me what was wrong with them, and I would do my best to find out and tell them. Now, they arrive having already done their own research. In their eyes, I'm just here to confirm what they already think they know.'

In 2007, Scott Haig, then an assistant clinical professor of orthopaedic surgery at Columbia University College of Physicians and Surgeons, published an essay in *Time* magazine titled 'When the Patient Is a Googler' that sent ripples of outrage through newly formed online medical communities. In it, Haig describes an appointment he recently conducted with 'Susan', a well-spoken, fit and attractive woman in her forties who is suffering from chronic knee pain. He already had his suspicions about her during their preparatory phone call, since he believes he can hear 'the soft click-click of the keyboard in the background' as she fact-checks his statements online in real time. In person, he finds everything about her obnoxious. Susan has brought her toddler with her to the clinic – presumably because she had no alternative – and Haig hates that the child 'dribbles chocolate milk from his sippy cup all over my upholstered chairs'. She has researched where he went to medical school and even read a recent paper that he has published. She also hits him with 'a barrage of excruciatingly well-informed questions' and, he feels sure, will be able to tell if he tries 'punting' her to another clinician because he doesn't want to treat her. If there is an element of being a doctor that requires performance – the confidence, the good bedside manner that soothes the patient – then Susan sees right through him, in other words.

Haig does admit that there is nothing wrong with trying to be well informed about your health or your choice of doctor, but something about the combination of Susan's confidence and her chosen research method (the internet) makes him lose all sense of proportion. He makes her background reading about his work sound like it is only just short of stalking. 'I was unnerved by how she brandished her information, too personal and just too rude on our first meeting,' he declares. He has sized her up instantly, he says, and knows that she will be a nightmare of a patient, utterly self-involved and full of complaints about conditions that will not show up on tests. Every doctor knows 'brainsuckers' like her and despises treating them. He writes yearningly about the 'non-compliant Bozos' who don't even want to know what is wrong with them and just trust their doctor to treat them, as well as how nice it is to treat engineers who are 'logical' about their health issues. He ends by lying to her, saying that he can't treat her problem (in the essay he asserts that he could do a good job if he chose) and recommending an alternative specialist – with whom, it turns out, she has already made an appointment. This is the final insult, of course. Susan has dared to consider other options for her treatment before even visiting Dr Haig. Truly, she is the 'queen, perhaps, of all Googlers'.

Much circulated and commented on – it was even covered in the *New York Times* – this essay polarised the emerging debate about the role that the internet could play in the future of medical care. Patient advocate groups roundly condemned Haig as pompous and entitled, suggesting that doctors who expressed such views were most likely threatened by what patients with access to up-to-date medical information might discover about the inadequacy of their physician's knowledge. This is certainly a reasonable reading of the essay; beneath all the sly prejudice,

Haig seems to be saying 'she thought she knew more than me, and that is not acceptable'. Then there were those inclined to be anxious about their health, who wrote earnestly that the new fashion for patients to research their illnesses wasn't part of some deliberate power grab, but rather a response to necessity. Just like the hypochondriacs of the eighteenth century, driven into the arms of the quacks because the mainstream doctors couldn't find anything wrong with them to treat, patients now go into consultations armed with sheaves of material printed off the internet in an attempt to make the case to their doctor that their need for medical treatment should be taken seriously. Other experts, though, dug their heels in alongside Haig, insisting that he was right to point out how unproductive it can be when a patient fires off statistics they have found on the internet in response to any treatment suggestion. More reasoned voices that tried to talk about how increased access to medical information could be used sensibly – perhaps if doctors were involved in curating the resources that patients used, for instance – were drowned out.

None of this put people off from using the internet to investigate their health issues, of course. Studies have consistently shown that for at least the last decade over eighty per cent of people use online resources for queries about health. The terminology used to describe these patients varies, from the more disparaging 'googler', who suffers from 'internet print-out syndrome', to the more neutral 'e-patient', 'health seeker' or exhibitor of 'online health information-seeking behaviour'. Just as with the many synonyms that have been tried out for 'hypochondria', some of these terms feel like they are too loaded with the expectation that the patient is being unreasonable in their desire to be better informed about their care. Interestingly, the one that has stuck in the small academic field around this topic actually imports and updates the millennia-old term. 'Cyberchondria' is the word that you will find in research papers about this even now, long after the internet has become an embedded part of every aspect of life, and it no longer seems strange or unreasonable to spend many hours sleuthing online about something before going to speak to a real person about it.

Not all people who casually type 'symptoms of brain cancer' into a search engine are cyberchondriacs, of course, just as not everybody who occasionally feels anxious about their headache lasting for three whole days is a hypochondriac. Cyberchondria manifests as repeated and escalating concerns about common symptoms, which in part occur as a result of searching and consuming information online. Hypochondria has changed yet again, keeping pace with this fundamental alteration in human lifestyle. It is still as slippery and quixotic as ever, though. Among the many stories I have been told while writing this book, there are several about someone who was dismissed by a doctor as a hypochondriac before being able to prove the validity of their symptoms with information they found on the internet. The woman who went to her doctor with chronic fatigue symptoms stands out to me; she was convinced she was in the early stages of fibromyalgia, but after an initial scan came back clear it took a lot of research and insistence on her part to secure the follow-up blood tests and examinations that ultimately confirmed the presence of the condition. Once a diagnosis vindicating the patient has been made, though, they are no longer an unreasonable cyberchondriac preferring the diagnosis of 'Doctor Google' over the real-life doctor sitting in front of them. After their research is proved correct, it is retrospectively reframed as due diligence and intelligent scepticism. The narrative of the illness is rewritten to support this new ending.

Cyberchondria is not just the excessive research suggested as a symptom by the *DSM-5*, though. It is also a function and feature of the metadata upon which the internet runs. Search engines are not neutral: they are commercial products designed and constantly tweaked to feed users more of the results they want so as to keep them on the page for longer. Our every click is monitored and analysed to train the algorithms that rank results. What experts call 'escalation' – the process by which a simple search for the probable causes of headaches becomes a deep dive into the prevalence of brain cancers in the searcher's age group – is aided by the very technology we're using to search. The more we jump from search terms about mild complaints to information about rare terminal conditions, the more likely it is that the search engine will rank those pages higher up the next time the search is performed, even if there is some element of weighting involved to push people towards more 'reputable' resources. Studies analysing millions of web pages accessed for medical queries show how even the design elements of search engines can push this escalation process onwards – those prompts that suggest endings to our sentences, for instance. Typing 'does headache mean . . .' into Google gives me the suggestions 'miscarriage', 'concussion' and 'brain tumour', which are all rather more serious issues than the far more common and likely causes of 'dehydration', 'stressed about work' and 'lack of fresh air'. The internet acts like a megaphone for a hypochondriac; I whisper my problem into it, and it is returned to me as an all-consuming shout. Distress and anxiety are what drive us to our screens in the first place, and what we find there then produces yet more distress and anxiety. A problem searched is a problem amplified.

*

The architecture of the internet, then, is built in such a way that it supports and even exacerbates our hypochondriac impulses. As we saw with the examples of Jerome K. Jerome and John O'Connell with their medical dictionaries, the exposure to a larger than expected amount of information about potential health problems can send the anxious mind spiralling far beyond the extent of the original fear. Both writers are exaggerating for comic effect, of course, but not by much. Something similar to their experiences with medical dictionaries happens when a cyberchondriac gets trapped in a never-ending spiral of increasingly doom-laden internet searches. The difference, though, is that Jerome's dictionary eventually comes to an end – 'there were no more diseases after zymosis', he records in great relief – but the scroll of the internet goes on forever. An app like TikTok provides the perfect conditions for trapping a cyberchondriac in this way. The slightest upwards flick of the thumb shows another video, and another, and another, each tailored by the algorithm to deliver more of what made you hover for longer over the last one. Experts working on online extremism and hate speech talk about something called the 'radicalisation pipeline', which they theorise can act as a pathway between more moderate and more extreme content. The same pattern can be posited for health-related content: the more interest a user shows in the discussion of a particular condition, the more posts they will be shown in that niche, and those recommended posts may well move from just those by qualified expects to also include amateur speculation and misinformation. A 2022 study that examined the hundred most popular videos about attention deficit hyperactivity disorder (ADHD) on TikTok classified over half of them as misleading, the majority of which were uploaded by people who were not qualified healthcare providers.

My particular online health vice is not data or definitions but anecdotes. That same study about the most popular ADHD TikToks showed that I am very far from being alone in this: of these videos, the ones with the highest engagement from other users described a personal experience or told a first-person story, rather than delivering more abstract or general information. Even though I am well aware of survivorship bias and the pitfalls of over-emphasising one inexpert individual's experiences at a population level, I can't seem to stop myself. When I'm worried about something, I find it comforting to seek out the stories of those who have experienced the same thing and lived to tell the tale. It can be dangerous, though. More than once I have become sucked in by a hypnotic account of a devastating diagnosis followed by a miracle cure and found myself on an unknown website browsing supplements with very long names before I come to my senses and have to put my phone in a drawer for a while. And of course, not all of these stories have the endings that I want, but that doesn't stop me surfing for the next one, and then the next. I'm like a gambler, always optimistic that the next one will be the big one, blowing on the dice to ensure that my lucky number comes up even though I know, deep down, that my breath means nothing at all.

It was during the height of the Covid pandemic and the consequent lockdowns in 2020 that TikTok exploded in popularity. With a large proportion of people suddenly working or studying from home and unable to socialise in person, the casual immediacy of the videos on the app helped to meet a need for interaction. It was especially attractive to young people – one survey found that the number of users aged fifteen to twenty-five grew by 180 per cent in the early months of 2020. By September of the following year, TikTok had a billion active users around the world and overtook all other social networks to become the most downloaded app of 2021. TikTok tends to be less hierarchal than other social media apps (any video, whether it comes from an established 'influencer' or a teenager in their bedroom, can go viral) and a more positive space. There are instances of bullying and hate, of course, but the app's architecture seems less adapted to spread them far and wide than that of other social networks. During lockdown, its endless loop of ever-present videos was comforting; while flicking upwards through people dancing, laughing, crying, cooking, cleaning, playing with animals and singing, we didn't have to think about what else was going on in the world. Of the many and varied types of content that emerged from this sudden influx of people with time on their hands, there is one that speaks particularly to the relationship between hypochondria and the internet. This involved people sharing details of their health conditions, especially ones with visible symptoms or behaviours that suit the short-form video medium, and discussing with followers how they adapt the details of everyday life to accommodate them. A whole subculture formed around Tourette's syndrome in particular, a condition characterised as a 'neurodevelopmental disorder' that can cause 'motor and vocal tics', such as involuntary twitching, eye rolling and outbursts of talking or shouting. Some of TikTok's Tourette's accounts quickly became popular, gathering millions of followers and a largely supportive community. Older Tourette's creators often make positive comparisons with the way they had to grow up decades ago, isolated and derided for symptoms that they did not understand. In the comments on these videos, people reported feeling validated by the non-judgemental way symptoms and experiences were shared; occasionally I would see someone say that they never realised what had been punished for 'being disruptive' could in fact be the result of a neurological disorder.

By March 2021, however, doctors and mental health specialists were reporting a marked increase in the number of children and adolescents – mostly girls, who ordinarily have far fewer instances of Tourette's than boys – presenting with tic symptoms, as well as more new cases of sudden and severe tic-like attacks. Many had no family history of Tourette's, which is also unusual since there is a genetic component to the disorder, with an estimated fifty per cent likelihood that a parent will pass it on to their child. Various causes were considered possible: the stress of the pandemic 'unmasking' an existing predisposition to tics, the change in routine and isolation necessitated by lockdown precautions, and exposure to social media videos in which tic-like symptoms were shown.

There is no test for Tourette's – a diagnosis is usually made if a number of common factors are present, such as a family history of the disorder, the onset of tics before the age of eighteen and the consistency of tic attacks for over twelve months. The sudden-onset cases that these girls were presenting with during the pandemic did not match most or indeed any of these conditions, and were thus categorised as a 'functional' illness. This is a relatively new concept in medicine, which seeks to describe conditions that would otherwise have been classified as somatic or 'medically unexplained'. It is a means of recognition without explanation: the word 'functional' is meant to indicate that the symptoms are considered 'real' – whatever that actually means – and do signify something going on in the body, even if tests cannot isolate a precise cause or pathology. They are evidence of something within finding an external release, even if we don't know what or why. The sudden appearance of these tics in teenage girls during Covid lockdowns was quickly identified as 'a partial component of functional neurological disorder'. The bigger question, however, was whether this was being caused by the consumption of tic-related content on social media.

The evidence for this was not long in coming. By the summer of 2021 papers were appearing that described the onset of 'TikTok tics' in dramatic terms as 'a pandemic within a pandemic' and 'an example of social contagion or mass sociogenic illness'. There were comparisons made to earlier reports of so-called social contagion in which psychosomatic symptoms like fainting and nausea seemed to be transmitted through social groups. In the Middle Ages, for example, there were reports of 'dancing mania' or 'St Vitus's Dance', in which entire groups of people, sometimes thousands at a time, began dancing erratically and apparently involuntarily, continuing until they were injured or collapsed from exhaustion. Various explanations have been proposed, including epilepsy and disorders of the nervous system, but it is most commonly understood as a form of mass hysteria, in which just seeing the symptoms of others was enough for someone else to 'catch' them. Something similar happened in the wake of the 1918 influenza pandemic too, when there were mass outbreaks of encephalitis lethargica, or 'sleepy sickness'. This involved a high fever and headaches as well as excessive sleeping, and even, in extreme cases, catatonia, a state in which someone is technically conscious but unable to respond to anything in their environment. There are plenty of other examples, many of them primarily experienced by young women, such as the mass fainting fits that are periodically reported as occurring in schools around the world.

Researchers entertained the possibility that TikTok was now turbocharging this mass-hysteria effect through the internet. By seeing peers and role models exhibit tics, viewers became more likely to develop them, either because of sug-gestibility, latent insecurity or a desire to share in the validation the original poster received online. The worldwide interest in this hypothesis and media reports will only have contributed to the effect, of course. Until 2020, these functional tic-like behaviours (or FTLBs, as they soon came to be called, because everything is more real when it has an official abbreviation) had accounted for a small fraction of referrals to tic disorder clinics. The new profusion of this specific disorder, along with the fact that a substantial majority of these patients reported watching tic influencers on TikTok and the similarity of the symptoms all around the world, allowed researchers to say with confidence that this was a condition at least partly triggered by watching it documented on the internet.

Was it a 'functional illness' though, or just hypochondria? I couldn't help whispering this question to myself as I watched all of this unfolding in my app and followed the accompanying scientific literature. I mean this with no judgement or derision – as I hope the preceding pages have made amply clear – but rather as a suggestion that the forces at play here are very similar to what has been called hypochondria in the past. The lack of so-called organic disease. The response to a collective trauma. The high incidence of co-morbidity with depression and anxiety. It fits. The mechanism by which FTLBs seem to spread could theoretically work for any kind of illness or several simultaneously; the stress caused by the pandemic could surely cause all kinds of problems, but for some unknown reason this phenomenon coalesced around Tourette's and tics specifically. There is a symbolic power to it, in the same way that medieval sufferers believed themselves to be made of glass, rather than ash or soil. The tics make possible the bodily expression of the fact that something is broken in the way that we expect young people to behave during a time of unprecedented crisis. Swearing, flailing limbs, shouting – these would usually be frowned upon or even punished. But in this form, they are carefully studied and validated by experts. In this way, the TikTok tics are the anti-glass delusion, a mark of how far we have come in the last several centuries. Rather than wishing to be invisible, these sufferers are taking up space and insisting on recognition in a way that I find admirable. Why should they keep calm and carry on? Look at us, they seem to say. We are not ok, and neither are you.

I would like to be able to tell you that after all the time spent prostrate inside the MRI machine, the answer to the baffling question of my intermittent vision problems was discovered, that they were able to pinpoint the vital missing piece needed to provide a unifying explanation for a disparate set of symptoms. In a world in which we have the technology to understand the previously secret workings of the human body, we assume that a scan, a test, an investigation will put an end to our uncertainty. And, after months of being confounded by unexplained and bizarre health events, I had come to feel that knowing would be better than not knowing, even if the prognosis was bad.

All the medical technology worked just as it should have done: those invisible eyes were able to see straight through me, capturing pictures of me in slices that the experts were able to examine. But, the scan revealed nothing of concern. This was the end of the road, diagnostically. It was a relief that the growth they had been searching for did not exist, but this simply ruled out one possible theory for the ongoing episodes. The technology the medical profession now has at its disposal for diagnosis offers the illusion of full knowledge, just as being connected to the internet tempts us to think that it has the answers to all our questions. But the body is still more opaque than we think, it retains its mysteries, especially when it comes to the way in which each individual experiences bodily sensation and pain.

There is no satisfying closure to this loop. I was given a small daily dose of a medication for low blood pressure, which reduced the number of episodes from several a week to just a few a year. I still take this pill every day, dutifully refilling the prescription every month, despite having no idea why I am doing so or what malfunction of my body it is treating. I used to request annual reviews of this medication with my GP, in a vain attempt to keep the search for a deeper cause going, but stopped after many years of identical meetings in which I was told slightly different versions of 'the pills are working, so let's not interfere'. Perhaps one day it will turn out that this medication is doing me harm in some hitherto unknown way, but for now it serves the purpose of suppressing something that cannot be explained, of holding my fears on this particular matter at bay.

8

The Mind–Body Problem

For months now, I have been haunted by the image of hypochondria as an enormous pendulum. Over the millennia, it has swung from being entirely a condition of the body, accelerating through the bottom of the arc where body and mind became blended and confused, and then momentum has carried it on up to the other side, where hypochondria exists only in our heads. The opposite of where we started. The end of the line; the pendulum can go no further. There, hypochondria received a new name – health anxiety – and joined a whole panoply of mental health conditions in the late twentieth century that were defined by just that: they were of the mind. Plenty of them have bodily components, such as body dysmorphia or obsessive compulsive disorder, which can manifest with repetitive behaviours that take the form of physical actions. But the starting point is the intangible mental processes that then influence the body, not the other way around.

The diagnosis of health anxiety occurs via an imperfect blend of art and science. After the patient has described how their mental state feels, their psychiatrist will use a combination of clinical observation, questionnaires and classification works like the *DSM-5* to find which condition or conditions best fit the symptoms and experience. For a long time, health anxiety was considered untreatable, but since the 1980s progress has been made. Treatment options vary according to diagnosis, but talking therapies in conjunction with drugs that alter the brain chemistry are a common combination. Short-term health anxiety, such as around a particular hospital visit or life event, can be treated with benzodiazepines – sedative drugs that work very quickly to slow down the nervous system and reduce feelings of anxiety and panic. Since these can be addictive or dangerous if taken for long periods, other pharmacological routes have been tested for long-term hypochondria sufferers.

There has been some success with a blend of CBT and selective serotonin reuptake inhibitors or SSRIs, a type of drug often used to treat depression. Both are aimed not at understanding why someone experiences health anxiety (whether that may be past trauma or a relationship to another condition), but rather at mitigating present symptoms and reframing the experience of them to reduce distress. Studies have consistently shown that antidepressants, especially when used in conjunction with CBT, cause a marked reduction in perceived symptoms and an improvement in overall wellbeing – in some cases this protocol performs up to sixty-seven per cent better than the placebo. For decades now, though, researchers have been lamenting the lack of a large-scale clinical trial investigating *why* antidepressants help with a condition that is widely agreed to be something other than depression. For now, all we can say is that higher serotonin levels seem to help the brain break out of hypochondriacal thought patterns and reduce the experience of unexplained symptoms. Treating the mind helps to treat the body.

A pendulum doesn't just swing once and stay still. It swings back, following the same path in reverse. And there are signs from the last fifteen years that the mind-only way of understanding mental health conditions may not be the ultimate answer, after all. The movement is small and slow, just a fraction of the pendulum's original arc, but it is happening. The body is returning.

In 2008, the US's National Institute of Mental Health included in its strategic plan something called 'the Research Domain Criteria Project' (RDoC). This laid out an ambition to find a new way of categorising mental health disorders based on detectable, observable behaviours and biological markers. This approach allows scientists to abandon the traditional categories in psychology, built up over decades of using subjective observations and patient surveys, and instead use tools like genetic tests and neurological imaging to tell one condition from another. Such a revolution in the diagnostic approach is long overdue. The reliability of purely psychiatric diagnosis techniques has been questioned since at least the 1960s. One study published in the *British Journal of Psychiatry* in 1974 found evidence of the 'obvious unreliability of psychiatric diagnosis' and observed that even when clinicians of similar background and training looked at the same patients, they were likely to come to different conclusions. Even with many decades of research and attempts to compile 'definitive' classifications of different mental health problems, and a growing awareness of the role played by prejudice or unconscious bias, the subjectivity of each human diagnostician still heavily influences the outcome.

It is in part to mitigate this problem that there is such interest in finding a biomedical underpinning for mental health diagnosis. But it is also because new discoveries in fields like genetics are beginning to make it seem possible. Scientists can now identify some cancers and types of diabetes, for instance, by looking at genetic markers; the ambition is to one day be able to do the same for mental health conditions that are currently only diagnosable based on the observable symptoms they cause. The opportunities for more precise and consistent diagnosis as well as earlier detection from such developments are clear, but this would also represent a major shift in how we conceptualise disease. If the RDoC, and similar international projects, do eventually lead to a blood test for schizophrenia, say, or a scan for health anxiety, can we really describe them as mental health conditions anymore? Diagnosis will only be made by minutely observing the body, perhaps even at a molecular level. The old idea of a division between mind and body will be completely swept away: everything that the mind perceives will have a detectable cause in the physical body. 'When I touch your skin and goosebumps lift, / it's your mind that surfaces there,' Wayne Miller writes in his poem 'Mind-Body Problem'. We think with our skin and move with our thoughts. There is no separation.

This biomedical approach brings us closer to the hypo-chondriac's ultimate dream: a definitive test for everything, including health anxiety itself. Imagine the immense relief a patient would feel if with just one tiny prick of the finger, they can put all their anxieties about their symptoms to rest using verifiable evidence from substances and processes within their body, if, almost immediately, a machine could spit out an answer like 'yes, you do have diabetes and this is how bad it is' or 'nothing going on here, you're worrying about nothing'. This is the utopian fantasy that home vitamin deficiency testing kits and fraudulent projects like Theranos were appealing to, without the science to back up their claims. Like so many, I am utterly enamoured of this idea that we could definitely tell when something is 'just health anxiety' and when it isn't. But as critics of the RDoC approach point out, this kind of testing is still the stuff of science fiction and people are experiencing mental health problems in the present, not the future. What we have now is largely still psychology and works like the *DSM* – but also a growing awareness of the way in which the body and the mind interact.

The human body is a reaction machine. Almost everything it does is a response to a stimulus or a change of some kind, whether that is a drop in the temperature outside or the growth of a tumour within. This is a relatively recent development in understanding: at the start of the nineteenth century, a cough or a fever was considered to be part of a disease, but by the start of the twentieth century it was considered to be evidence of the healthy body's response to a disease. We cough to clear our airways of mucus or irritants that may do lasting harm if allowed to remain, and a temporary rise in temperature is part of an immune response that seeks to make the body an inhospitable environment for pathogens. These are ways that a resilient body survives. Rather than being signs of decline, they are usually signs of hope. I didn't grasp this until I was given a course of chemotherapy so toxic that it utterly destroyed my immune system. My medical team explained that it was now vital that they wake me every four hours to perform basic checks to keep me safe. I absolutely despised this regime, since it meant that I could never sleep for longer than about three hours at a time and thus, on top of everything else, felt constantly exhausted, but it was essential. I no longer had any white blood cells that would organise a protective response to an invading infection or cause easily visible signs of a fightback like sweating or aches. Unless I was minutely monitored, by the time I physically felt that something was wrong with my responseless body, it would be too late to save me.

This is the framework within which we place hypochondria today, harking back to its origins early in our evolutionary journey as a way to increase the chances of survival in a world full of dangers. Like other kinds of protective behaviours, hypochondria is a response to a threat, a way of coping. Reactions to mental stressors generally fall into one of two kinds: pathological consequences, such as when post-traumatic stress disorder alters the way some parts of the brain function, and coping mechanisms, with which the nervous system adapts and triggers involuntary behaviours to maintain a functional level of mental health. Hypochondria is this latter kind of defence mechanism, sometimes called an 'immature defence', because it is not ultimately productive or helpful in the long term. It channels anxiety and fear into a certain sphere – health – that can make it feel productive, but it remains a destructive force for the sufferer as they get stuck in the never-ending loop of uncertainty it provides. The choice of defence mechanism is unconscious; nobody deliberately selects hypochondria over something more measured such as affiliation or the drive to seek support from others. A complex web of genetic, social and environmental factors determines how the body reacts to stressful and traumatic circumstances.

Even though the likes of the nineteenth-century French neurologist Jean-Martin Charcot worked extensively on the idea of traumatic memories that continue to haunt decades later, for much of the following century this idea was not fashionable. Freud and the psychoanalysts were far more interested in the interplay and conflict of different kinds of mental instinct – the ego, the id, the libido, and so on – and this remained the dominant paradigm for mental illness until the fallout from the World Wars forced a reconsideration. The mass trauma experienced on the battlefields of the twentieth century meant that millions of people survived the fighting only to spend the rest of their lives suffering from mental and physical symptoms like amnesia, hallucination, tics, mood disorders and, in more extreme cases, what was described as 'functional paralysis'. A variety of different terms were used for this mysterious condition, including shell shock, war neurosis and neurasthenia, until the waves of traumatised personnel returning to the US from Vietnam in the 1960s and 1970s finally prompted more systematic and scientific studies of why this was happening. By 1980, 'post-traumatic stress disorder' (PTSD) had become an officially diagnosable condition, included in the third edition of the *DSM*, and the idea that past trauma could continue to have an impact on the mind and body was well on the way to becoming a basic tenet of neuroscience and psychology.

Today, there is wide acceptance of the idea that 'the body keeps the score' of past trauma that the mind is holding on to – a book of that title by the psychiatrist and trauma researcher Bessel van der Kolk has sold millions of copies and spent over a hundred weeks atop the *New York Times* bestseller list. 'The human response to psychological trauma is one of the most important public health problems in the world,' van der Kolk wrote in a journal article over twenty years ago. Military service is now just one of the arenas where PTSD is a recognised risk; accidents, sexual assaults, disasters, family violence and more are all potential sites of trauma. Physical, or somatic, symptoms with no clear explanation are a common accompaniment to past trauma. A large study of military veterans with PTSD conducted in 2021 found that almost sixty per cent of those with a full PTSD diagnosis experienced at least one, and often several, such symptoms, including digestive problems, nausea, headaches and chronic joint or back pain. Similar results have been found in children and adults with trauma from other circumstances, such as sexual assault, who end up reporting 'more medical visits, more major illnesses and hospitalizations' than control groups.

Recent popular culture has comprehensively imbibed this idea too. In the first episode of the BBC's *Sherlock* produced in 2010, Dr John Watson has what the viewer is told repeatedly is a 'psychosomatic limp'. A military doctor recently invalided home from service in Afghanistan, his difficulties walking and standing are strongly emphasised in the first half hour of the show. We see him giving truculent answers about it in a consultation with his therapist, struggling to walk downstairs, dropping into an armchair with a guttural sigh of relief at no longer having to bear his own weight on his painful leg. We settle into the idea that this is how his trauma is expressing itself. Easily visible physical symptoms like this are not an uncommon way for screenwriters to depict PTSD – having somebody shake or limp or experience involuntary flashbacks is more obviously visual and dramatic than if they just move through the world normally while all of the trouble rages inside their head. It's a palatable way of portraying something for which many people have instinctive negative assumptions; that someone is faking it, malingering or deliberately monopolising medical resources. Focusing attention on a so-called worthy sufferer is a common trick too. Watson, with his status as a military veteran and a doctor, is an easy object of sympathy. He is otherwise able-bodied, slim, white and clearly desperate to be active and employed. He has one brief outburst of anger about his limitations – '*Damn* my leg!' – for which he immediately apologises. An interesting exercise to apply to portrayals of imaginary illness, I find, is to contemplate how they would be written if the sufferer was someone for whom society had less instinctive compassion.

Watson's worthiness established, then comes a scene where Holmes and Watson are on foot, closing in on a suspect in a car. They dash out of the restaurant where they have been keeping watch, and in the rush of the pursuit Watson leaves his walking stick behind. A few frenetic minutes of chasing follows, with Watson performing some quite remarkable parkour-like feats including jumping from roof to roof and jogging down a tight spiral staircase. *Come on, John*, Sherlock yells from time to time, as if his partner is an able-bodied man dragging his heels, rather than a wounded veteran who could barely walk a few minutes before. They miss out on collaring the suspect, and it isn't until they are back at home that John realises he no longer has his stick, or any need of it. The exciting combination of the danger and his fully occupied mind has freed him from the traumatic memories and anxiety that were causing the limp, which he previously believed to be the result of a gunshot wound. It seems like a miracle, of the 'take up your bed and walk' kind, until Sherlock starts laughing – he has deliberately engineered the chase so as to prove to John that his limp was all in his head, and it has worked.

Traumatic memories remain so vivid and impactful, capable of making chemical and even physical changes to the body, because of how the brain processes the experience. The primary stress responders in the brain are the amygdala, hippocampus and prefrontal cortex – together, they deal with the emotional intensity of an experience and its context. The amygdala, sometimes called the brain's smoke detector, triggers stress hormones and nervous system actions in response to perceived danger that can be life-saving: fight or flight responses like increased heart function and blood pressure. When the system is out of balance, though, this response might be called up when it is not needed; a sudden movement in the corner of the eye will recall the original trauma, for instance, and the body will leap into stress mode before other areas of the brain can assess whether this is justified. Living with an amygdala in constant overdrive results in an exhausting level of constant hypervigilance, and can ultimately cause the mind and body to dissociate – nobody can function with their smoke alarm going off all the time. The insula, the area of the brain that processes input from the rest of the body and sends information about potential danger to the amygdala, begins to shut down. The only way to survive is for mind and body to separate. Alexithymia is one consequence of this, a phenomenon in which a person can no longer feel what emotions they are experiencing or what is upsetting them. Without this information, sensation gets pushed into their body instead: their anger might surface as joint pain, their sadness as digestive issues, and so on.

Before this trauma response was widely understood, these patients would seek medical attention for their physical ailments in the normal way, only for doctors to tell them that there was nothing causing these symptoms – an unhelpful diagnosis for someone already struggling with a disconnect between mind and body. When he began his work with military veterans in the 1970s, van der Kolk observed that the waiting rooms of his medical colleagues were full of old men who had served in the Second World War and were now presenting with a complex cocktail of unexplained physical issues, whereas the younger Vietnam veterans, more familiar with the new developments in mental health, were being treated by psychiatry. These elderly veterans scored highly on tests for PTSD and trauma-related conditions too – their pain had been expressing itself in the only way they knew. In the end, it is the changes the trauma sets off that cause the body long-term harm, rather than the trauma itself. 'Like a splinter that causes an infection, it is the body's response to the foreign object that becomes the problem more than the object itself,' van der Kolk explains. Long after the original trauma has vanished, the body is still experiencing it, fighting an invisible enemy that nobody else can see.

Hypochondria is not PTSD, but it shares some of the same characteristics, and the two can go together. Many people with PTSD experience some combination of health anxiety and somatic symptom disorder, but not everybody with health anxiety has PTSD. The disconnection between mind and body, the mysterious symptoms that originate in the mind but express themselves in the body, the hypervigilance to bodily disorder – these and more are common experiences of both problems. The relationship that hypochondria has with traumatic health events also suggests a link with trauma issues. In many cases, the symptoms of hypochondria begin after a close friend or family member has suffered or died with a serious illness. There is also evidence that what psychologists call 'adverse childhood experiences' are linked to a greater rate of health anxiety in adulthood. This might be a serious medical condition experienced at a young age, or a factor like family violence, caregiver substance abuse or neglect. The resulting trauma impacts the way in which the person appraises their feelings of illness, predisposing them to be uncertain and negative about any physical sensations.

About six months into the Covid pandemic, I developed terrible problems with sleep. I had always been a deep, almost voracious sleeper, never able to get enough rest even if I slept for eight, nine, ten hours a night. Suddenly, though, I could barely keep my eyes closed for three. I would fall asleep and fall straight into a vivid dream based on some twisted medical fear of mine: the memory of a pelvic bone biopsy I had once would replay, for instance, except they forget to give me the anaesthetic this time, or I am rushed into surgery, cut open and left there awake and alone in the operating theatre because all the doctors have been called away by a 'real' emergency while I lie there listening to the sound of my own blood slowly pooling on the floor beneath the table. A favourite one was the replay of the procedure that had extracted eggs from my eighteen-year-old ovaries before I received a cancer treatment that had a high chance of destroying my fertility. That became an alien-egg-harvesting nightmare that I had a lot. Each time, I would jolt awake as if I really had been stabbed with a scalpel, and sleep would not come again that night. When I was awake, I berated myself for not being able to overcome the power of these memories from so long ago, which I had never been aware of as a problem before. This, combined with my ambient daily anxiety that I might be infected by a deadly respiratory virus any second, made my sleeplessness even worse. The slightest sound or bodily discomfort could keep me awake all night, both desperate to sleep and terrified of what I might experience in my dreams if I did. As anyone who has suffered from long-term insomnia will know, a chronic lack of sleep ruins everything else: it magnifies all existing problems. Every tickle in the throat or impetus to sniff – and there are a lot of them; I have fairly severe allergies – heralded what was surely the beginning of the end.

After a few months navigating overwhelmed mental health services and being offered a lot of pre-recorded online courses in CBT to do alone, I ended up with a therapist who specialised in responses to trauma of all kinds – I was initially attracted to her because her bio said she had worked extensively in war zones. My problems, by contrast, were insignificant, I felt, and thus should pose no challenge for her. She proposed that I try one of the therapies she offered for trauma-related problems, eye movement desensitisation and reprocessing (EMDR). This is a therapy that combines revisiting the trauma memories while engaging in a form of bilateral stimulation, usually by repeatedly moving the eyes from left to right or tapping alternate sides of the chest. It was first proposed in 1987 by American psychologist Francine Shapiro, who had noticed during a walk in the park that moving her eyes rapidly from side to side provided some relief from the distressing memories she was contemplating. Shapiro evolved a protocol that involves recalling memories while moving the eyes, with a therapist guiding the patient through their recollections and the associations that come up with them until the initial trauma ceases to evoke such distress.

I was sceptical; I still am. We used a bar with an LED that moved from side to side along it to guide my eye movements, and I superstitiously chose the colour green for it, holding on to its associations with progress and forward movement. At the start, it felt too close to a ritual to be scientific, and indeed EMDR has been criticised as a pseudoscience or even a form of modern-day 'mesmerism'. It makes me think of Jean-Martin Charcot at his Parisian hospital in the nineteenth century, insisting that his hysterical patients were fundamentally more susceptible and thus treatable via hypnotism. However, there is also a substantial body of experts – including Bessel van der Kolk – who are very enthusiastic about the efficacy of EMDR as a way of allowing patients to revisit traumatic memories without retraumatising themselves, and reintegrate them into their proper context as an event that occurred in the past, thus removing that disabling feeling of ever-present danger.

Some studies, including van der Kolk's own, show moderate or good patient outcomes from EMDR. It has been partially adopted as an official treatment, with caveats: the American Psychiatric Association 'conditionally recommends' it as a treatment for PTSD, and the National Institute for Health and Care Excellence in the UK also endorses its use for PTSD – although not for other mental health issues like grief or depression – while noting that there is 'limited evidence' upon which to assess its effectiveness.

An EMDR session begins with a discussion of the specific trauma memory to be processed and how it makes the client feel. As the therapist prompts me to begin speaking each time, she turns on the light, and I track its movement along the bar with my eyes, side to side. In one session, I worked on the moment I was told I had cancer, from which so many of my anxieties flow. I am told to conjure up the memory, the heart of the trauma. I think of the consulting room, of the doctor across the desk from me, of the nurse standing at his elbow, the solid presence of my mother in the chair next to me. He delivers the news. My mother droops and slides off the chair in a faint. The nurse springs forward to help her. I remain behind with the doctor and ask him if I'm going to die.

After about fifteen seconds of thinking and bouncing my eyes side to side in rhythm with the shifting light the therapist interrupts gently, saying 'OK, what are you feeling?' I try to clear my mind and describe whatever is welling up. The first time, it is anger. I'm furious that I'm in that room receiving that diagnosis, and I'm also furious that I'm in this room, eyes bouncing from side to side as I relive it. After a brief acknowledgement of this response, I'm directed to resume the eye movements and think about the anger. This continues, the interruptions, the descriptions, the injunctions to continue.

It's like playing a word association game except with the worst moments of my life.

Sometimes I know as soon as I resume moving my eyes what the next memory or sensation I describe is going to be, and I just let it marinate as I flick my gaze back and forth, waiting for the prompt to speak it aloud. At other times, there is only blankness and I'm surprised at what comes out when I start speaking. Occasionally, I get too far away from the locus of the trauma, the moment of diagnosis, and the therapist tells me to go back there, to restart. She is quietly authoritative, encouraging me to keep going but not lifting the pressure to face the hard things for a second.

As the process continues, I lose any sensation of time passing. The memories are grim, but the feeling of total focus is almost pleasant. It is rare these days that I manage to spend over an hour so concentrated on one thing, and it satisfies an itch in my brain somewhere that I was barely aware of. At some point, I start crying and only notice I'm doing it when the tears start dripping off my chin. The therapist puts a box of tissues on the sofa next to me and I briefly pause to wipe my face.

Gradually, a common thread emerges from the welter of disjointed images and impressions. I am furious about the diagnosis, but not in the 'why me?' way I had always assumed. I'm not angry about being told I have cancer, but at the way I was conditioned to react. I didn't scream, or cry, or faint, or really express my fear or horror in any way. I sat quietly on the chair after my mother had been taken away to recover and tried to ask the doctor sensible questions about what would happen next. My true reaction, the emotional tornado whipped into being by his words, was instantly and instinctively contained and ignored, pushed down into my body to await moments of weakness as I dropped off to sleep over a decade later. Only now, feeling a bit absurd while I follow the path of the green light back and forth with my eyes, was I probing the extent of it.

Afterwards, for about twenty-four hours, my brain feels like a raw prawn that has recently been plucked from its protective shell. I feel like I have a bruise, a tender patch somewhere, except it is not anywhere on my body I can inspect. Connections have been made that cannot be unmade now and I have been scraped clean of something, like wood that has been stripped of old paint to reveal a fresh new surface beneath. The sensation gradually fades over the coming days. I cautiously attempt to sleep through the night again, braced for the dreams and confused when they don't come. I still have trouble sleeping sometimes when I'm especially anxious about something, but I have not had the vivid dreams of past medical experiences once since this session, and I'm a little better at controlling my panic. I have also applied this same technique to other sources of trauma in my past, such as my teenage experiences with fertility treatments, with similarly positive results. The memories are still there and I can summon them to think about if I want to, but they belong to the past now. In the present, I am someone else.

There is another emerging technique that offers a different way of rebalancing the relationship between mind and body. Pain neuroscience education (PNE) is a cognitive technique aimed at helping patients with chronic pain, often in the musculo-skeletal system and without an identifiable cause, to reframe their understanding so that they experience less discomfort. It developed from work being done in the field of physical therapy and aims to put a stop to 'pain catastrophising'. This is a thought loop in which an anxious patient tends to magnify the pain they are experiencing and feel helpless to do anything about it. They can become locked into this pattern, unable to think about anything other than their pain, which then takes on a dominant role in their life. This can even happen in anti-cipation of pain; someone who has been injured a lot in the past, for instance, might have anxiety about it that leads them to overestimate how much something that hasn't yet happened might hurt in the future. One common presentation is with a painful injury that has been healed but is still causing discom-fort long after doctors can no longer detect any tangible reason for it to be doing so.

As part of PNE, a patient is given scientific information by their doctor about how pain works: the neurobiology that governs how the brain interprets sensations and sends signals about them around the body. Some aspects of the protocol focus on reframing the way the patient thinks and talks about their bodily experience, encouraging the use of words like 'sen-sation' or 'discomfort' instead of the more loaded 'pain'. Rather than talking about not being able to do things 'because of the pain', they are encouraged to see what they can do 'despite the pain'. A major factor in this process is being able to imagine separating the self from the sensation. In one account, a chronic pain sufferer who found great relief from PNE wrote that it helped to 'visualize my pain as a person or a monster, screaming for attention, whom I needed to firmly, gently reassure – not take directions from'. If someone has lived with mysterious or undiagnosed pain for a long time, their need to make meaning out of something so difficult and so open-ended often leads to them recasting memories and life events in light of their relation to their pain to the point that their core narrative is tightly bound up with it. Gradually diminishing the role that pain plays in identity can help. In 2021, a study was conducted on women with endometriosis – a gynaecological condition for which there is no cure and that often goes undiagnosed for years, in which endometrial tissue grows outside the womb, causing bleeding, pain and cysts. The results revealed that those who constructed narratives with the illness less central to their identity were more likely to experience better mental health, less anxiety about their condition and even potentially less pain. Like hypochondria, pain can overwhelm the story that you tell about yourself, and the body holds on to it to make sure that the story continues.

This work is at the frontier of the mind–body problem, in my opinion. PNE takes the mental and physical aspects of pain together as one and harnesses the same emotional power of suggestion and expectation that drives the nocebo effect to decouple the body from pain that is mostly or entirely experienced in the mind. It is worth noting that it does not work for everybody, though. There are many positive examples cited in the clinical literature where people have been able to diminish their intake of opioid painkillers because of PNE, for example, or reduce their healthcare costs. But it isn't a miracle cure that removes all pain sensations overnight, and every study that tries to measure its impact includes details of participants who saw little or no change from the treatment. The same is true of EMDR – it works for some, me included, but not for everybody. That perfect, universal cure that the hypochondriac daydreams of does not exist.

Writing about hypochondria goes against the narrative grain that we have been conditioned to follow when it comes to telling stories about illness. If somebody were to submit my own experiences to me as an outline for a future article, I would send it back to them with comments about the lack of a clear arc and the need for a clever callback to the main theme near the end.

It lacks structure. Sensations are there, and then they are not there. I can only write through it, as it happens, and let go of that niggling desire for a closure that never comes.

Even after all of my medical and hypochondriacal adventures, I still find myself easily slipping back into an absolutist frame of mind that I recognise from my childhood, before cancer introduced me to all the myriad complexities held within the apparently simple ideas of 'treatment' and 'cure'. When I fall down and cut myself, I put on a plaster and then I will be fine again. Part of me persists in believing, absurdly, that this is how all injuries and illnesses should work. But almost nothing is so simple and so linear. The five years that I have worked on this book have seen some extreme low points for me, some triggered by external circumstances like the Covid pandemic, and others prompted by the memories I was unearthing for my writing. The account of all the shifting, nameless ailments I have experienced while worrying about finishing this book would fill a volume of their own. I worried throughout, too, that I was doing something wrong by sharing an unfinished story: I am still the same anxious, health-obsessed person I was when I began. The perfectionist in me thought I needed to complete the process and tick off the trauma before I could share it. I was perpetually braced for a moment of absolute catharsis, a good ending, that has yet to arrive.

If I had waited for that, though, this book would not exist. If there is a personal lesson I have extracted from my years immersed in this, it is that there are no perfect narrative arcs or neat endings, no matter how much our instincts tell us to seek them out. I used to think of illness and health anxiety as things that happened in addition to my life, in a separate sphere that I could duck in and out of – this compartmentalisation was a big part of how I dealt with having cancer while also finishing school and getting a university degree without taking any breaks at all. What I know now is that there is no such separation: they are both aspects of my existence that will remain with me for as long as I am alive. I have spent a lot of time worrying about whether, by revealing this part of myself to the public, I am making hypochondria too much part of my identity. Is my perpetual health anxiety a foregone conclusion if it is on display like this? An unanswerable question.

During an early discussion about this book, someone asked me whether I would be giving it a happy ending. 'Perhaps you could talk about the cure for hypochondria?' she said, hopefully. 'End on an up, you know.' I think I made a joke in the moment, probably something about how it would make for a better story if I died from one of my imaginary ailments. I mentioned that Spike Milligan has a line in Irish engraved on his headstone: *Dúirt mé leat go raibh mé breoite*, 'I told you I was sick.' His widow had to fight with the church to get something so apparently flippant permitted on hallowed ground; the compromise was putting it in a language that few visitors to Winchelsea in East Sussex will speak. Everything about hypochondria is there in those few words; it is silly, dramatic, terrifying, disturbing, bewildering, contradictory. To fear illness is to fear death. Some treatment programmes for hypochondria begin by asking the sufferer if they are willing to be mortal. What a question. If hypochondria is rooted in a search for certainty, there is no greater certainty than that. I don't think hypochondria will ever leave us, either. Doubt is human, and so is fear, and so is hope. In fact, the continued presence of hypochondria ultimately reassures me. We have been trying to make sense of this for thousands of years, and we are still trying.

It was a line from John Donne that finally helped me to let go of the idea that I need to be less fragile, less breakable, less conscious of my every twinge and scrape. 'Variable, and therefore miserable condition of man! This minute I was well, and am ill, this minute,' he wrote at the opening of his *Devotions*. Scratched onto the page 400 years ago while he was in the grip of a terrible fever, those words encapsulate how I feel every day. I am ill and I am well. I am still here.

Notes

Introduction: The People Made of Glass

p. 9   '... *suspended in darkness*': Nunberg, H., and Federn, E. (eds.), *Minutes of the Vienna Psychoanalytic Society, Vol. II: 1908–1910* (International Universities Press, Inc., 1967), p. 210

p. 10   '*the bible of psychiatry*': https://www.scientificamerican.com/article/dsm-5-update/

p. 10   '*extensive worries about health*': *DSM-5*, p. 314

p. 10   '*easily alarmed about personal health status*': Ibid., p. 315

p. 11   *The authors of one study*: Bailer, J., Kerstner, T., Witthöft, M., et al., 'Health anxiety and hypochondriasis in the light of DSM-5', Anxiety, Stress, & Coping, 29.2 (2016) 219–39. https://doi.org/10.1080/10615806.2015.1036243

p. 11   '... *hypochondriasis and health anxiety*': Ibid. p. 16

p. 12   '*the persistent and unwarranted belief* ...': Definition from *Oxford English Dictionary*

p. 13   '... *not fully explained by a general medical condtion*': *DSM-IV*, p. 445

p. 13   '*the stigmatising hypochondriasis label*': Fink, P., Ørnbøl, E., Toft, T., et al., 'A new, empirically established hypochondriasis diagnosis', American Journal of Psychiatry, 161.9 (2004) 1680–91. https://doi.org/10.1176/appi.ajp.161.9.1680

p. 13   *coinage from 1988*: Oyebode, F., *Sims' Symptoms in the Mind: An Introduction to Descriptive Psychopathology* (Baillière Tindall, 1988), pp 171–96

p. 14   '... *weak or sickly constitution*': Definition from *Merriam-Webster*

Dictionary, https://www.merriam-webster.com/dictionary/valetud inarian

p. 14   *'somatoform disorder'*: Mayou, R., Kirmayer, L. J., Simon, G., et al., 'Somatoform disorders: time for a new approach in DSM-V', American Journal of Psychiatry, 162.5 (2005) 847–55. https://doi. org/10.1176/appi.ajp.162.5.847

p. 14   *one expert earnestly concludes*: Starcevic, V., 'Somatoform disorders and DSM-V: conceptual and political issues in the debate', Psychosomatics, 47.4 (2006) 277–81. https://doi.org/10.1176/appi. psy.47.4.277

p. 15   *according to some experts*: Belling, C., *A Condition of Doubt* (OUP, 2012), p. 13

p. 20   *'Constantine said ...'*: Kolb, P. (ed.), *Marcel Proust: Selected Letters 1880–1903* (University of Chicago Press, 1983), p. 205

p. 22   *'It is in sickness ...'*: Proust, M., *The Guermantes Way*, translation by Scott Moncrieff, C. K., and Kilmartin, T. (Modern Library, 2003), p. 404

p. 24   *the Greek physician Galen of Pergamon*: He was born Greek but moved to Rome and was most famous for practising there.

p. 24   *'... in order not to be broken'*: from *Galen on the Affected Parts*, Book 3, Ch. 20, quoted in translation from Pormann, P. E., 'New fragments from Rufus of Ephesus' "On Melancholy"', The Classical Quarterly, 64.2 (2014) 653. https://www.jstor.org/stable/43905603

p. 24   *fifth and sixth centuries*: Pormann, P. E., *'Rufus of Ephesus On Melancholy'* (Mohr Siebeck, 2008), p. 33

p. 26   *King Charles VI*: Speak, G., 'An odd kind of melancholy: reflections on the glass delusion in Europe (1440–1680)', History of Psychiatry, 1.2 (1990) 191–206. https://doi.org/10.1177/0957154X9000100203

p. 26   *a completely different person*: Gabel, L. C. (ed.), *Memoirs of a Renaissance Pope: the Commentaries of Pius II*, translation by Gragg, F. A. (Smith College Studies in History, 1951), p. 425

p. 26   *'... which humanity has been assailed'*: de Cervantes Saavedra, M., *The Exemplary Novels of Cervantes*, translation by Kelly, W. K. (Duke Classics, 2015), p. 231

p. 27   *a royal physician*: André du Laurens, doctor to Philip II of Spain and Henri IV of France

p. 27   *in which he languished*: Speak, G., p. 193

p. 27   *'the most learned professors of medicine and philosophy'*: de Cervantes Saavedra, M., p. 233

p. 27   '*. . . Like the glass in the window*' Shepherd, V., *A History of Delusions: The Glass King, a Substitute Husband and a Walking Corpse* (Oneworld, 2022), p. 181

p. 28   *the doubt itself*: Belling, C., p. 1

p. 29   *the phrase* licenciado vidriera: Definition from *Diccionario de la lengua española*

p. 31   *humans 'are meaning makers'*: Hale, B., *The Evolution of Bruno Littlemore* (Atlantic Books, 2011), p. 184

Chapter 1: The Origins of the Ancient Malady

p. 35   *Studies at the genetic level*: Fumagalli, M., Sironi, M., Pozzoli, U., et al., 'Signatures of environmental genetic adaptation pinpoint pathogens as the main selective pressure through human evolution', PLOS Genetics 7.11 (2011) e1002355. https://doi.org/10.1371/journal.pgen.1002355

p. 35   *avoid contact with them altogether*: Schaller, M., and Park, J. H., 'The behavioral immune system (and why it matters)', Current Directions in Psychological Science, 20.2 (2011) 99–103. https://doi.org/10.1177/0963721411402596

p. 35   *limiting the risk of infection*: Kurzban, R. and Leary, M. R., 'Evolutionary origins of stigmatization: the functions of social exclusion', Psychological Bulletin, 127.2 (2001) 187–208. https://doi.org/10.1037/0033-2909.127.2.187

p. 36   *fears of specific animals*: Ware, J., Jain, K., Burgess, I., et al., 'Disease-avoidance model: factor analysis of common animal fears', Behaviour Research and Therapy, 32.1 (1994) 57–63. https://doi.org/10.1016/0005-7967(94)90084-1

p. 36   *other individuals and animals*: Hart, B. L., 'Biological basis of the behavior of sick animals', Neuroscience & Biobehavioral Reviews, 12.2 (1988) 123–37. https://doi.org/10.1016/S0149-7634(88)80004-6

p. 36   *this behavioural immune system*: Kanageswaran, N., Nagel, M., Scholz, P., et al., 'Modulatory effects of sex steroids progesterone and estradiol on odorant-evoked responses in olfactory receptor neurons', PLOS ONE, 11.8 (2016) e0159640. https://doi:10.1371/journal.pone.0159640

p. 36   *A study carried out in 2021*: Leschak, C. J., Hornstein, E. A., Byrne Haltom, K. E., et al., 'Ventromedial prefrontal cortex activity differentiates sick from healthy faces: associations with inflammatory responses and disease avoidance motivation', Brain, Behavior, and Immunity, 100 (2022) 48–54. https://doi. org/10.1016/j.bbi.2021.11.011

p. 37   *vmPFC plays a role in regulating the amygdala*: Motzkin, J. C., Philippi, C. L., Wolf, R. C., et al., 'Ventromedial prefrontal cortex is critical for the regulation of amygdala activity in humans', Biological Psychiatry, 77.3 (2015) 276–84. https://doi.org/10.1016/j. biopsych.2014.02.014

p. 38   *even on a subconscious level*: Neuberg, S. L., Kenrick, D. T., and Schaller, M., 'Human threat management systems: self-protection and disease avoidance', Neuroscience & Biobehavioral Reviews, 35.4 (2011) 1042–51. https://doi.org/10.1016/j.neubiorev.2010.08.011

p. 38   *'threat-signalling cue'*: Ibid.

p. 39   *a 2016 study*: Hedman, E., Lekander, M., Karshikoff, B., et al., 'Health anxiety in a disease-avoidance framework: investigation of anxiety, disgust and disease perception in response to sickness cues', Journal of Abnormal Psychology, 125.7 (2016) 868–78. https:// doi.org/10.1037/abn0000195

p. 39   *'hyperactive disease avoidant mechanisms'*: Ibid., p. 869

p. 39   *'. . . the dreaded illness'*: Rachman, S., 'Health anxiety disorders: a cognitive construal', Behaviour Research and Therapy, 50.7–8 (2012) 502–12. https://doi.org/10.1016/j.brat.2012.05.001

p. 40   *patched with a fragment*: Smith, L., 'The Kahun gynaecological papyrus: Ancient Egyptian medicine', Journal of Family Planning and Reproductive Health Care, 37.1 (2011) 54–5. https://doi. org/10.1136/jfprhc.2010.0019

p. 40   *'Examination of a woman . . .'*: Kahun Gynaecological Papyrus, Column 1, Lines 25–27.
Translation: https://www.ucl.ac.uk/museums-static/digitalegypt/ med/birthpapyrus.html

p. 41   *a thousand years earlier*: Breasted, J. H., *The Edwin Smith Surgical Papyrus Published in Facsimile and Hieroglyphic Transliteration with Translation and Commentary in Two Volumes* (University of Chicago Press, 1930), Vol. 1, p. xiii

p. 43   *'medical and magical throughout'*: Dawson, W. R., *Magician and Leech: A Study in the Beginnings of Medicine with Special Reference to Ancient Egypt* (Methuen, 1929), p. 5

p. 43   *'subtle mysterious disturbances'*: Bryan, C. P., and Smith, G. E., *Ancient Egyptian Medicine: The Papyrus Ebers* (Ares, 1930), p. xviii.

https://babel.hathitrust.org/cgi/pt?id=coo.31924073200077&view=1up&seq=5

p. 44   *holy dung*: Ibid., p. 61

p. 48   *painful cocktail of mysterious illnesses*: Lambert, W. G., *Babylonian Wisdom Literature* (OUP, 1960), p. 21

p. 48   '*Debilitating Disease* ...': Ludlul bēl nēmeqi, Tablet 2, Line 50. Translation by Lambert, W. G., in *Babylonian Wisdom Literature* (Clarendon, 1960)

p. 48   *Babylonian courtier Šubši-mešrê-Šakkan*: Geller, M. J., *Ancient Babylonian Medicine: Theory and Practice* (Wiley-Blackwell, 2010), p. 73

p. 48   '*My complaints* ...': Ludlul bēl nēmeqi, Tablet 2, Lines 108–11.

p. 49   *only discovered in 2008*: I am grateful to Professor Maria Grazia Masetti-Rouault of l'École Pratique des Hautes Études, Sorbonne, for sharing details of this as yet unpublished study

p. 50   '... *since childhood*': Geller, M. J., p. 74

p. 50   *a healthy body and mind*: Kleisiaris, C. F., Sfakianakis, C., and Papathanasiou, I. V., 'Health care practices in ancient Greece: The Hippocratic ideal', Journal of Medical Ethics and History of Medicine, 7.6 (2014). https://pubmed.ncbi.nlm.nih.gov/25512827/

p. 50   *wombs being 'displaced'*: Hanson, A. E., 'Hippocrates: 'Diseases of Women 1', Signs: Journal of Women in Culture and Society, 1.2 (1975) 567–84. https://doi.org/10.1086/493243

p. 51   *targeted and effective care*: Bonadonna, G., 'Historical review of Hodgkin's disease', British Journal of Haematology, 110.3 (2000) 504–11. https://doi.org/10.1046/j.1365-214

Chapter 2: All Disease Begins in the Gut

p. 54   '... *some other perturbation*': *The Tusculan Disputations of Cicero*, revised and corrected by Main, W. H. (W. Pickering, 1824), p. 186

p. 54   aegritudo: Crocq, M.-A., 'A history of anxiety: from Hippocrates to DSM.' Dialogues in Clinical Neuroscience, 17.3 (2015) 319–25. https://doi.org/10.31887/DCNS.2015.17.3/macrocq

p. 55   '*hypochondrion*': Hippocrates, Case IV, Epidemics I

p. 55   '*Jaundice supervening* ...': *Aphorisms Of Hippocrates*, translation by Marks, E. (Collins, 1817), p. 93

p. 55   '... *distention of the hypochondrium*': Ibid., p. 119

p. 55   '... *relieved by fever*': Ibid., p. 133

p. 56   '*... almost two inches*': Sheldon, G., *A History of Deerfield, Massachusetts* (Greenfield, Mass: Press of E. A. Hall & Co., 1895), p. 448

p. 56   *passing away at the age of eighty-three*: https://www.geni.com/people/Deacon-Samuel-Field/6000000006727980641

p. 57   '*... in the entire Corpus ...*': Nuland, S. B., *Doctors: The Biography of Medicine* (Knopf, 2011), p. 4

p. 58   *the community at large*: von Staden, H., 'The discovery of the body: human dissection and its cultural contexts in ancient Greece', Yale Journal of Biology and Medicine, 65.3 (1992) 223–41. https://www.ncbi.nlm.nih.gov/pmc/articles/PMC2589595/

p. 58   *Diocles of Carystus*: Conti, A. A., and Paternostro, F., 'Anatomical study in the Western world before the Middle Ages: historical evidence', Acta Bio Medica Atenei Parmensis, 90.4 (2019) 523–5. https://doi.org/10.23750/abm.v90i4.8738

p. 58   *augmented by Egyptian texts*: von Staden, H., p. 225

p. 59   "*To him medicine owes ...*": Garrison, F. H., *An introduction to the history of medicine* (W. B. Saunders, 1917) p. 82

p. 61   '*... one of the body's tissues*': Weinberg, R. A., *One Renegade Cell: How Cancer Begins* (Basic Books, 1998), p. 12

p. 62   *Robert Dudley and his wife*: Gregory, P., *The Virgin's Lover* (Simon & Schuster, 2005)

p. 62   *foreshadowing of the cancer*: Patel, S. K., and Jacobs, R., 'The suspicious demise of Amy Robsart', Iowa Orthopaedic Journal, 23 (2003) 130–1. https://www.ncbi.nlm.nih.gov/pmc/articles/PMC1888393/

p. 66   '*people-shadows*': http://www.alexeytitarenko.com/cityofshadows

p. 66   '*... the juices flowed*': Lieberman, J. J., and Lieberman, S. J., 'A short history of quackery and byways in medicine', The American Biology Teacher, 37.1 (1975) 39–43. https://doi.org/10.2307/4445041

p. 68   '*... individual and environment*': Arikha, N., *Passions and Tempers: A History of the Humors* (Ecco, 2007), p. xviii

p. 69   *a confirmation of the theory*: Ibid., p. 80

p. 70   *an excess of black bile*: Hippocrates, Aphorisms 6:23. http://classics.mit.edu/Hippocrates/aphorisms.6.vi.html

p. 70   '*aversion to food ...*': Hippocrates, Epidemics II. http://classics.mit.edu/Hippocrates/epidemics.2.ii.html

p. 70   '*... identifiable illnesses*': Arikha, N., p. 116.

p. 71   '*That part of the soul ...*': Plato, *Timaeus*, Sect. 3, Ch. 38

p. 72   '*like a napkin* …': Ibid.

p. 72   '*For just as darkness* …': Pormann, P. E., *Rufus of Ephesus On Melancholy* (Mohr Siebeck, 2008), p. 285

p. 72   '… *hypochondriac and flatulent*': Ibid.

p. 74   '*a limited vocabulary of subjective sensations*': Belling, C., *A Condition of Doubt* (OUP, 2012), p. 69

p. 76   '*microbiota–gut–brain axis*': Cryan, J. F., O'Riordan, K. J., Cowan, C. S. M., et al., 'The microbiota–gut–brain axis', Physiological Reviews, 99.4 (2019) 1877–2013. https://doi.org/10.1152/physrev.00018.2018

p. 76   *depression*: Pinto-Sanchez, M. I., Hall, G. B., Ghajar, K., et al., 'Probiotic *Bifidobacterium longum* NCC3001 reduces depression scores and alters brain activity: a pilot study in patients with irritable bowel syndrome', Gastroenterology, 153.2 (2017) 448–59. e8. https://doi.org/10.1053/j.gastro.2017.05.003

p. 76   *anxiety*: Campbell, S. A., Needham, B. D., Meyer, C. R., et al., 'Safety and target engagement of an oral small-molecule sequestrant in adolescents with autism spectrum disorder: an open-label phase 1b/2a trial', Nature Medicine, 28.3 (2022) 528–34. https://doi.org/10.1038/s41591-022-01683-9

p. 76   *degenerative neurological diseases*: Gotkine, M., Kviatcovsky, D., and Elinav, E., 'Amyotrophic lateral sclerosis and intestinal microbiota-toward establishing cause and effect', Gut Microbes, 11.6 (2020) 1833–41. https://doi.org/10.1080/19490976.2020.1767464

Chapter 3: Sharp Belchings and Windy Melancholy

p. 79   *the cost of this can be very high*: Fink, P., Ørnbøl, E., and Christensen, K. J., 'The outcome of health anxiety in primary care. A two-year follow-up study on health care costs and self-rated health', PLOS ONE, 5.3 (2010) e9873. https://doi.org/10.1371/journal.pone.0009873

p. 79   *census data*: https://www.census.gov/library/publications/2022/demo/p60-278.html

p. 79   *Black people are far more likely to be uninsured*: https://www.census.gov/content/dam/Census/library/publications/2022/acs/acsbr-012.pdf

p. 80   *Santiago Levín*: Nicoletti, P. M., 'Hypochondria is a lot more than being worried about getting sick', Vice, 22 September 2021

p. 83   *Donne's 'astonishing alertness to disease'*: Scarry, E., 'Donne: but yet the body is his booke', in Scarry, E. (ed.), *Literature and the Body: Essays on Populations and Persons* (Johns Hopkins University Press, 1990), p. 72, Note 6

p. 88   *'achingly fashionable'*: Shepherd, V., *A History of Delusions: The Glass King, a Substitute Husband and a Walking Corpse* (Oneworld, 2022), p. 119

p. 89   *'logical dissection'*: Definition from *Oxford English Dictionary*

p. 89   *James Boswell*: Boswell, J., *Life of Dr Johnson* (1791), Vol. I, p. 339

p. 90   *'... analyst of the psyche'*: Dell, F. and Jordan-Smith, P. (eds.) *The Anatomy of Melancholy* (Tudor Publishing Company, 1938) p. 16

p. 90   *Jennifer Radden*: Radden, J., *Melancholic Habits* (OUP, 2016)

p. 103   *'seized with a convulsion'*: Matthews, B., *Molière: His Life and His Works* (Hardpress, 2013), p. 317

p. 106   *'my faithful muse'*: https://www.newyorker.com/cartoons/bob-mankoff/hypochondria-faithful-muse

p. 106   *'My father was a doctor ...'*: https://www.latimes.com/lifestyle/story/2020-04-10/comic-marc-maron-explains-how-to-be-a-hypochondriac-during-a-pandemic

p. 107   *'ridiculous'*: Ibid.

p. 107   *while swimming alone in a pool*: Bloom, C., *Leaving a Doll's House* (Virago Press, 1996), p. 184

p. 108   *'... on closer terms with my insurance plan ...'*: Ibid., p. 220

p. 108   *'... distinguish epidemiology from anti-Semitism'*: https://forward.com/culture/397567/is-there-really-such-a-thing-as-jewish-anxiety/

p. 108   *Centuries of persecution*: https://www.huffpost.com/entry/im-not-a-hypochondriac-im_b_3664073

Chapter 4: Spirits, Vapours and Nerves

p. 113   *'the animal within'*: http://classics.mit.edu/Plato/timaeus.html

p. 113   *'like some animal inside an animal'*: Gilman, S. L., King, H., Porter, R., et al., *Hysteria Beyond Freud* (University of California Press, 1993), p. 26

p. 113   *'voracious, predatory, appetitive, unstable'*: Ibid., p. 107

p. 114   *'from the bottom of his belly upwards'*: Willis, T., and Pordage, S., *An Essay of the Pathology of the Brain and Nervous Stock in Which Convulsive Diseases Are Treated of* (1681), p. 37. https://quod.lib.umich.edu/e/eebo/A66496.0001.001/1:3.5?rgn=div2;submit=

Go;subview=detail;type=simple;view=fulltext;q1=histerical #hl3

p. 115   '*... as one egg is to another*': Sydenham, T., *The Works of Thomas Sydenham, M. D.*, translation from the Latin edition of *Dr. Greenhill with a Life of the Author* by Latham, R. G. (1848), Vol. II, p. 85

p. 115   '*... these two affections*': Foucault, M., *Madness and Civilization: A History of Insanity in the Age of Reason*, translation by Howard, R. (Vintage Books, 1988), p. 145

p. 116   *Henry Joly*: Joly, H., *Discours d'une estrange et cruelle maladie hypocondriaque venteuse, qui a duré onze ans: Accompagnée de l'hystérique passion, avec leurs noms, causes, signes, accidents terribles, & leurs remèdes* (Catherine Niverd, 1609)

p. 116   '*hysteria-hypochondriasis*': Veith, I., 'On hysterical and hypochondriacal afflictions', Bulletin of the History of Medicine, 30.3 (1956) 233–40. https://www.jstor.org/stable/44450567

p. 117   '*... the bad influence of the uterus*': Foucault, M., p. 213

p. 119   *pain is subjective*: https://www.jpain.org/article/S1526-5900(21) 00035-3/fulltext#seccesectitle0031

p. 120   *four times as likely to die in childbirth*: https://www.theguardian.com/ society/2021/nov/11/black-women-uk-maternal-mortality-rates

p. 120   *2.6 times as likely in the US*: https://www.cdc.gov/nchs/data/hestat/ maternal-mortality/2021/maternal-mortality-rates-2021.htm

p. 122   '*mumbo jumbo*': Gilman, S. L., King, H., Porter, R., et al., p. 236

p. 124   *good or evil*: Foucault, M., p. 139

p. 129   *vapours arising from the spleen and liver*: Joly, H., Ibid.

p. 129   '*... almost all Diseases*': Purcell, J., *A Treatise of Vapours, or Hysterick Fits: The Second Edition, Revis'd and Augmented* (Edward Place, 1707), p. 2

p. 130   '*... the nerves and the muscles*': Foucault, M., p. 160

p. 130   '*... amuse the People with words*': Arnaud, S., *On Hysteria: The Invention of a Medical Category Between 1670 and 1820* (University of Chicago Press, 2015), p. 18

p. 132   '*... I couldn't even see my own eyes*': https://www.vanityfair.com/ hollywood/2018/01/tiffany-haddish-interview-in-the-spotlight

Chapter 5: The Rise and Rise of the Quack

p. 133   *One study from 2011*: Tyrer, P., Cooper, S., Crawford., M., et al., 'Prevalence of health anxiety problems in medical clinics', *Journal of Psychosomatic Research*, 71.6 (2011) 392–4. http://doi.org/10.1016/j. jpsychores.2011.07.004

p. 133 *another from ten years before*: Nimnuan, C., Hotopf, M. and Wessely, S., 'Medically unexplained symptoms: an epidemiological study in seven specialities', Journal of Psychosomatic Research, 51.1 (2001) 361–7. http://doi.org/10.1016/s0022-3999(01)00223-9

p. 134 *'The Paradox of Health'*: Barsky, A. J., 'The paradox of health', New England Journal of Medicine, 318.7 (1988) 414–8. https://doi. org/10.1056/NEJM198802183180705

p. 135 *'the Rich, the Lazy, the Luxurious, and the Unactive'*: Porter, R. (ed.), *George Cheyne: The English Malady* (1733), Tavistock Classics in the History of Psychiatry (Tavistock/Routledge, 1991) p. 28

p. 135 *'... exquisite and voluptuous Manner'*: Ibid., p. 28

p. 136 *'... his bodily Organs'*: Ibid., p. 29

p. 136 *'... class and standing'*: Rousseau, G. S., *Nervous Acts: Essays on Literature, Culture and Sensibility* (Palgrave Macmillan, 2004), p. 256

p. 136 *'... be hyppish, be nervous, be bilious, be rich'*: Ibid., p. 255

p. 136 *'These men going naked ...'*: Burton, R., *Anatomy of Melancholy*, Memo II, Subsect. III

p. 137 *'... a victim of vapors ...'*: Arnaud, S., *On Hysteria: The Invention of a Medical Category Between 1670 and 1820* (University of Chicago Press, 2015), p. 31

p. 139 *'The hysteric and hypochondriac ...'*: Rush, B., 'Inquiry into the natural history of medicine among the Indians of North-America and a comparative view of their diseases and remedies with those of the civilized nations', read before the American Philosophical Society, Philadelphia, 4 February 1774, p. 49

p. 140 *'... poor indigent man ...'*: Baur, S., *Hypochondria: Woeful Imaginings* (University of California Press, 1989), p. 26

p. 140 *... a hot branding iron to the skin*: Risse, G. B., *New Medical Challenges during the Scottish Enlightenment* (Brill, 2005), p. 27. https://doi.org/10.1163/9789004333000

p. 141 *his physician beating him*: Speak, G., 'An odd kind of melancholy: reflections on the glass delusion in Europe (1440–1680)', History of Psychiatry, 1.2 (1990) 191–206. https://doi. org/10.1177/0957154X9000100203

p. 141 *'... creature of his own brain'*: Risse, G. B., p. 21

p. 141 *'... indifferent living'*: Ibid., p. 22

p. 142   '... *self-imposed immaturity*': Kant, I., *What is Enlightenment?* (1784)

p. 143   '... *hypochondriac region*': Moore, J., *Medical Sketches: in Two Parts* (Printed for A. Strahan and T. Cadell in the Strand, 1786), p. 253

p. 143   '... *harbinger of disease*': Ibid., p. 254

p. 143   '... *the greatest insult*': Ibid., p. 255

p. 144   '*prescribing for imaginary complaints* ...': Ibid., p. 21

p. 146   *Ancient Rome*: Mattern, S. P., 'Physicians and the Roman imperial aristocracy: the patronage of therapeutics', Bulletin of the History of Medicine, 73.1 (1999) 1–18. https://doi.org/10.1353/bhm.1999.0038

p. 146   '... *false or fake remedies*': Definition from *Oxford English Dictionary*

p. 146   *salves for cysts*: Jameson, E., *A Natural History of Quackery* (Michael Joseph, 1961)

p. 147   '... *advertising his own concocted medicines* ...': Strathern, P., *Quacks, Rogues and Charlatans of the RCP* (Little, Brown, 2016), p. 16

p. 147   *cold, wet phlegm*: Gross, R. A., 'A brief history of epilepsy and its therapy in the Western Hemisphere', Epilepsy Research, 12.2 (1992) 65–74. https://doi.org/10.1016/0920-1211(92)90028-R

p. 147   '*empowered*': Lepere, I., 'Inside Mexico's temazcals: how the ancient Aztec healing ritual taught me self-reliance'. https://www.flashpack.com/solo/travel/mexico-temazcal-ritual/

p. 148   '... *two middle Fingers of the Right-hand*': Hall, J., *Select Observations on English Bodies of Eminent Persons in Desperate Diseases* (1679), pp. 23–4. https://ota.bodleian.ox.ac.uk/repository/xmlui/bitstream/handle/20.500.12024/A45063/A45063.html?sequence=5&isAllowed=y

p. 148   *powdered mummy*: da Silva Veiga, P. A., *Health and Medicine in Ancient Egypt: Magic and Science* (University of Michigan Press, 2009). https://doi.org/10.30861/9781407305004

p. 149   '*If a rhetorician* ...': Plato, Gorgias, Vol. 3, translation by Lamb, W. R. M. (Harvard University Press, 1925), p. 291

p. 150   *ancient yet contemporary story*: 'Fake psychiatrist Zholia Alemi who forged medical degree jailed', BBC News. https://www.bbc.co.uk/news/uk-england-lancashire-64797676

p. 151   *lose the entire contents of their stomach*: Strathern, P., p. 47

p. 152   '*The Pills consist of Snails*': Ibid., p. 59.

p. 153   '*an age of pills and potions*': King, S. in Curth, L. H. (ed.), *From Physick to Pharmacology: Five Hundred Years of British Drug Retailing* (Routledge, 2017), p. 166

p. 153　'*... rude and credulous populace*': Strathern, P., p. 13

p. 155　'*have it set by the fools ...*': Corley, T. A. B., 'Mapp [Née Wallin], Sarah (Bap. 1706, d. 1737), bone-setter', Oxford Dictionary of National Biography, Online (Oxford University Press, 2009). https://doi.org/10.1093/ref:odnb/56037

p. 156　'*... Knowledge is experience*': Strathern, P., p. 21

p. 156　*Thomas Hobbes*: Ibid., p. 34

p. 159　'*Nervous and hypochondriacal complaints ...*': Porter, R., *Quacks: Fakers and Charlatans in Medicine* (Tempus, 2000), p. 158.

p. 160　*around £50 today*: The National Archives, Currency converter: 1270–2017. https://www.nationalarchives.gov.uk/currency-converter/

p. 163　'*cult of invalidism*': Dijkstra, B., *Idols of Perversity: Fantasies of Feminine Evil in Fin-de-Siècle Culture* (OUP, 1988), p. 23

p. 163　'*consumption ... is a flattering malady*': King, C., *The Brontës Life and Letters Vol II* (Hodder and Stoughton, 1908), p. 23

p. 170　'*medical faith*': Howe, L. C., Goyer, J. P., and Crum, A. J., 'Harnessing the placebo effect: Exploring the influence of physician characteristics on placebo response', Health Psychology, 36.11 (2017) 1074–82. https://doi.org/10.1037/hea0000499

p. 170　'*a paper in* The Lancet': Graves, T. C., 'Commentary on a case of hystero-epilepsy with delayed puberty', The Lancet, 196.5075 (1920) 1134–5. https://doi.org/10.1016/S0140-6736(01)00108-8

p. 171　*double-masked placebo-controlled study*: Fallon, B. A., Petkova, E., Skritskaya, N., et al., 'A double-masked, placebo-controlled study of fluoxetine for hypochondriasis', Journal of Clinical Psychopharmacology, 28.6 (2008) 638–45. https://doi.org/10.1097/JCP.0b013e31818d21cf

p. 171　*between twenty and forty per cent*: https://www.drugs.com/article/placebo-effect.html

p. 172　'*semi-placebos*': Justman, S., 'Placebos in the clinic', Journal of the Royal Society of Medicine, 106.6 (2013) 208–9. https://doi.org/10.1177/0141076813489969

p. 172　*A 2020 study*: Guevarra, D. A., Moser, J. S., Wager, T. G., et al., 'Placebos without deception reduce self-report and neural measures of emotional distress', Nature Communications, 11.1 (2020) 3785. https://doi.org/10.1038/s41467-020-17654-y

Chapter 6: All in My Head

p. 176   '... *meaning in suffering*': Charon, R., 'Narrative medicine: a model
for empathy, reflection, profession, and trust', Journal of the
American Medical Association, 286.15 (2001) 1897. https://doi.
org/10.1001/jama.286.15.1897

p. 179   '*The exact opposite of the mind's power* ...': Kant, I., *The Conflict of
the Faculties/Der Streit der Facultäten*, translation by Gregor, M. J.
(Abaris Books, 1979), p. 187

p. 180   '... *mental occupation of thinking* ...': Ibid., p. 199

p. 185   *In a 1987 interview* ...': https://bordercrossingsmag.com/article/
style-and-radical-will

p. 189   *Sir John Hill*: Belling, C., *A Condition of Doubt* (OUP, 2012), p. 46

p. 191   '*a series of paradoxes without coherence*': Rousseau, G., *The Notorious
Sir John Hill: The Man Destroyed by Ambition in the Era of Celebrity*
(Lehigh University Press, 2012)

p. 192   *Alexander Pope*: Brownell, M. R., '"Like Socrates": Pope's art of
dying', Studies in English Literature, 1500–1900, 20.3 (1980) 407.
https://doi.org/10.2307/450288

p. 192   '... *a dose of salts*': Extracts from a diary of Lord Byron, 1821. https://www.
lordbyron.org/monograph.php?doc=ThMoore.1830&select=AD1821

p. 192   '... *the most usual causes of hypochondria*': Falret, J.-P., *De
l'Hypochondrie et du suicide* (1822), p. 444 (author's translation)

p. 192   '... *her skin was scaly like that of a carp* ...': Ibid. p. 416

p. 194   '... *tormented by day and by night*': Janet, P., *Les médications
psychologiques*, 3 Vols. (Société Pierre Janet, 1984)

p. 194   '*epitome of neurosis*': Baur, S., *Hypochondria: Woeful Imaginings*
(University of California Press, 1989), p. 29

p. 194   *Mrs A*: Freud, S., *The Complete Letters of Sigmund Freud to Wilhelm
Fliess, 1887–1904*, translation by Masson, J. M. (Belknap Press.
1986) p. 15

p. 195   '... *arises from his sexual life*': Ibid., p. 110

p. 195   '... *being in love with one's own illness*': Nunberg, H., and Federn, E.
(eds.), *Minutes of the Vienna Psychoanalytic Society, Vol. III: 1910–1911*
(International Universities Press, Inc., 1962), p. 243

p. 195   '... *suspended in darkness*': Nunberg, H., and Federn, E. (eds.),
Minutes of the Vienna Psychoanalytic Society, Vol. II: 1908–1910
(International Universities Press, Inc., 1967), p. 210

p. 195   *perceived as diseased*: Freud, S., *A General Introduction to
Psychoanalysis* (Boni & Liveright, 1920), p. 363

p. 195   '*pure forms of true neurosis*': Ibid., p. 339

p. 195   '*The symptoms of an actual neurosis*': Ibid., p. 336

p. 196   '*unanalysable*': Baur, S., p. 29

p. 196   '... *a beaten man*': Freud, S., *The Complete Letters* ..., p. 84

p. 199   '... *excessive fear of death* ...': Starcevic, V., and Noyes Jr., R. *Hypochondriasis and Health Anxiety: A Guide for Clinicians* (OUP, 2014), p. 27

p. 199   *studies measuring the attitudes towards death*: Noyes, R., Stuart, S., Longley, S. L., et al., 'Hypochondriasis and fear of death', The Journal of Nervous and Mental Disease, 190.8 (2002) 503–9. https://doi.org/10.1097/00005053-200208000-00002

p. 205   '*Life is first boredom, then fear* ...': Larkin, P., 'Dockery and Son', from *Whitsun Weddings* (Faber, 1964)

p. 206   *looked older than T. S. Eliot*: https://thelondonmagazine.org/essay-the-joys-of-depression-the-glamour-of-gloom-bishop-and-larkin-by-jeffrey-meyers/

p. 206   '*clenched irritation*': Motion, A., *Philip Larkin: A Writer's Life* (Gardners Books, 1994), p. 80

p. 206   '*a male chauvinist*': Ibid., p. 83

p. 208   *letters to Monica*: Larkin, P., *Letters to Monica*, ed. Thwaite, A. (Faber, 2010), p. 278

p. 210   '... *mother-fixation*': Larkin, P., *Required Writing: Miscellaneous Pieces 1955–1982* (Farrar Straus Giroux, 1984)

p. 213   *Emma, his devoted daughter*': Bartlett, N., *Jane Austen: Reflections of a Reader* (2021), p. 108. https://doi.org/10.11647/OBP.0216

p. 215   '*raise the emotional temperature* ...: Fergus, J., '"My sore throats, you know, are always worse than anybody's:": Mary Musgrove and Jane Austen's art of whining', Jane Austen Society of North America. https://jasna.org/persuasions/printed/number15/fergus.htm?

p. 215   '*chiefly in her head*': Letter from Jane Austen to her sister Cassandra, 8–11 April 1805

p. 215   '... *a liver disorder*': Letter from Jane to Cassandra, 18 December 1798

p. 215   '*a lifelong hypochondriac*': Bartlett, N., p. 93

p. 216   '... *vaguely defined invalidism*': Ibid., p. 60

p. 216   '*putrid fever*': https://mh.bmj.com/content/31/1/3

p. 217   '*two or three chairs*': Austen-Leigh, J. E., *A Memoir of Jane Austen* (Folio, 1989), p. 147

p. 218   '*... savage attack on hypochondria?*': Tomalin, C., *Jane Austen: A Life* (Penguin, 2012) p. 265

p. 218   '*... in His own good time*': Ibid., p. 282

Chapter 7: We Know Too Much

p. 224   *depressed brain activity*: Charles, A. C., and Baca, S. M., 'Cortical spreading depression and migraine', Nature Reviews Neurology, 9.11 (2012) 637–44. https://doi.org/10.1038/nrneurol.2013.192

p. 226   '*considered normal*': Wilhelmsen, I., 'Hypochondriasis or health anxiety', in *Encyclopedia of Human Behavior* (Elsevier, 2012), pp. 385–91. https://doi.org/10.1016/B978-0-12-375000-6.00197-X

p. 226   *One interesting study*: Herrmann, D. J., 'Know thy memory: the use of questionnaires to assess and study memory', Psychological Bulletin, 92.2 (1982) 434–52. https://doi.org/10.1037/0033-2909.92.2.434

p. 227   *Issy Pilowsky's Whiteley Index*: Pilowsky I., 'Dimensions of hypochondriasis', The British Journal of Psychiatry, 113.494 (1967) 89–93. https://doi.org/10.1192/bjp.113.494.89

p. 227   *Hypochondriasis Yale-Brown Obsessive-Compulsive Scale*: Fergus, T. A., Kelley, L. P., and Griggs, J. O., 'Examining the Whiteley Index-6 as a screener for DSM-5 presentations of severe health anxiety in primary care', Journal of Psychosomatic Research, 127 (2019) 109389. https://doi.org/10.1016/j.jpsychores.2019.109839

p. 229   '*..."the worried well"*': Gray, D. P., Dineen, M., and Sidaway-Lee, K., 'The worried well', British Journal of General Practice, 70.691 (2020) 84–5. https://doi.org/10.3399/bjgp20X708017

p. 230   *only heightens their anxiety*: O'Malley, P. G., Jackson, J. L., Santoro, J., et al., 'Antidepressant therapy for unexplained symptoms and symptom syndromes', The Journal of Family Practice, 48.12 (1999) 980–90. https://pubmed.ncbi.nlm.nih.gov/10628579/

p. 230   *so-called benign remedies*: Barsky, A. J., 'The patient with hypochondriasis', New England Journal of Medicine, 345.19 (2001) 1395–9. https://doi.org/10.1056/NEJMcp002896.

p. 239   '*... We are all little fairies*': Green J., *The Anthropocene Reviewed* (Dutton, 2021) p. 220

p. 241   *Multiple studies from the last decade*: Waterman, L. Z., and Weinman, J. A., 'Medical student syndrome: fact or fiction? A cross-sectional study', JRSM Open, 5.2 (2014) 204253331351248. https://doi.org/10.1177/2042533313512480; Katarzyna, S., Furgał,

N., Szczepanek, D., et al., '"Medical student syndrome" – a myth or a real disease entity? Cross-sectional study of medical students of the Medical University of Silesia in Katowice, Poland', International Journal of Environmental Research and Public Health, 18.18 (2021) 9884. https://doi.org/10.3390/ijerph18189884

p. 243   '... *assume elephantine proportions*': O'Connell, J., *I Told You I Was Ill: Adventures in Hypochondria* (Short Books, 2006), p. 31

p. 244   *'evil twin*': Glick, M., 'Placebo and its evil twin, nocebo', The Journal of the American Dental Association, 147.4 (2016) 227–8. https://doi.org/10.1016/j.adaj.2016.02.009

p. 244   *Dr Walter Kennedy*: Kennedy, W. P., 'The nocebo reaction', Medical World, 1961 Sep;95 (1961) 203–5.

p. 244   *One early trial from 1968*: Luparello, T., Lyons, H. A., Bleecker, E. R., et al., 'Influences of suggestion on airway reactivity in asthmatic subjects', Psychosomatic Medicine, 30.6 (1968) 819–25. https://doi.org/10.1097/00006842-196811000-00002

p. 245   *A recent review*: Haas, J. W., Bender, F. L., Ballou, S., et al., 'Frequency of adverse events in the placebo arms of COVID-19 vaccine trials: a systematic review and meta-analysis', JAMA Network Open, 5.1 (2022) e2143955. https://doi.org/10.1001/jamanetworkopen.2021.43955

p. 246   *A 2016 Norwegian study*: Berge, L. I., Skogen, J. C., Sulo, G., et al., 'Health anxiety and risk of ischaemic heart disease: a prospective cohort study linking the Hordaland Health Study (HUSK) with the Cardiovascular Diseases in Norway (CVDNOR) project', BMJ Open, 6.11 (2016) e012914. https://doi.org/10.1136/bmjopen-2016-012914

p. 246   *a figure ... so eye-catchingly high*': https://www.theguardian.com /science/2016/nov/03/worried-well-more-risk-heart-disease-research-finds

p. 247   *the nocebo effect*: Pan, Y., Kinitz, T., Stapic, M., et al., 'Minimizing drug adverse events by informing about the nocebo effect – an experimental study', Frontiers in Psychiatry, 10 (2019) 504. https://doi.org/10.3389/fpsyt.2019.00504

p. 247   *in a positive rather than negative way*: Faasse, K., Huynh, A., Pearson, S., et al., 'The influence of side effect information framing on nocebo effects', Annals of Behavioral Medicine, 53.7 (2019) 621–9. https://doi.org/10.1093/abm/kay071

p. 248   *'research their suspected disease excessively ...*': DSM-5, p. 317

p. 248   *Much of the nocebo literature*: B., Herbert, 'The nocebo effect: history and physiology', Preventive Medicine, 26.5 (1997) 612–15. https://doi.org/10.1006/pmed.1997.0228

p. 248   *retired to his bed and died*: Griesinger, G. A., *Biographische Notizen über Joseph Haydn* (Biographical Notes on Joseph Haydn), Facsimile edition with afterword & notes by Krause, P. (VEB Deutscher Verlag für Musik, 1979), p. 45

p. 249   *In a 1961 study*: Weisman, A. D., and Hackett, T. P., 'Predilection to death: death and dying as a psychiatric problem', Psychosomatic Medicine, 23.3 (1961) 232–56. https://pubmed.ncbi.nlm.nih.gov/13784028/

p. 250   *'When the Patient is a Googler'*: https://content.time.com/time/health/article/0,8599,1681838,00.html

p. 251   *even covered in the* New York Times: A doctor's disdain for medical 'Googlers', 19 November 2007. http://well.blogs.nytimes.com/2007/11/19/a-doctors-disdain-for-medical-googlers/

p. 252   *use online resources for queries about health*: The 2006 Pew Internet and American Life Project; Bujnowska-Fedak, M. M., Waligóra, J., Mastalerz-Migas, A. (2019). 'The internet as a source of health information and services'. in Pokorski, M. (ed.) *Advancements and Innovations in Health Sciences*. Advances in Experimental Medicine and Biology, Vol. 1211 (Springer, 2019). https://doi.org/10.1007/55842019396

p. 253   *consuming information online*: Definition from White, R. W., and Horvitz, E., 'Cyberchondria: studies of the escalation of medical concerns in web search', ACM Transactions on Information Systems, 27.4 (2009) 1–37. https://doi.org/10.1145/1629096.1629101

p. 254   *What experts call 'escalation'*: Ibid.

p. 255   *the 'radicalisation pipeline'*: Ribeiro, M. H., Ottoni, R., West, R., et al., 'Auditing radicalization pathways on YouTube', in Proceedings of the 2020 Conference on Fairness, Accountability, and Transparency (presented at *FAT '20: Conference on Fairness, Accountability, and Transparency*, Barcelona, Spain: ACM, 2020), pp. 131–41. https://doi.org/10.1145/3351095.3372879

p. 255   *A 2022 study*: Yeung, A., Ng, E., and Abi-Jaoude, E., 'TikTok and attention-deficit/hyperactivity disorder: a cross-sectional study of social media content quality', The Canadian Journal of Psychiatry, 67.12 (2022) 899–906. https://doi.org/10.1177/07067437221082854

p. 256 *one survey*: https://www.statista.com/statistics/1207831/tiktok-usage-among-young-adults-during-covid-19-usa/

p. 257 *the most downloaded app of 2021*: https://blog.apptopia.com/worldwide-and-us-download-leaders-2021

p. 257 *'motor and vocal tics'*: https://tourette.org/about-tourette/overview/

p. 258 *By March 2021*: Heyman, I., Liang, H., and Hedderly, T., 'COVID-19 related increase in childhood tics and tic-like attacks', Archives of Disease in Childhood, 106.5 (2021) 420–1. https://doi.org/10.1136/archdischild-2021-321748

p. 258 *a genetic component to the disorder*: https://www.cdc.gov/ncbddd/tourette/riskfactors.html

p. 258 *tics in teenage girls*: Heyman, I., Liang, H., and Hedderly, T., pp. 420–1

p. 259 *'a pandemic within a pandemic'*: Olvera, C., Stebbins, G. T., Goetz, C. G., et al., 'TikTok tics: a pandemic within a pandemic', Movement Disorders Clinical Practice, 8.8 (2021) 1200–5. https://doi.org/10.1002/mdc3.13316

p. 259 *There were comparisons*: Forsyth, R. J., 'Tics, TikTok and COVID-19', Archives of Disease in Childhood, 106.5 (2021) 417. https://doi.org/10.1136/archdischild-2021-321885

p. 260 *tic disorder clinics*: Pringsheim, T., Ganos, C., McGuire, J. F., et al., 'Rapid onset functional tic-like behaviors in young females during the COVID-19 pandemic', Movement Disorders, 36.12 (2021) 2707–13. https://doi.org/10.1002/mds.28778

p. 260 *triggered by watching it . . . on the internet*: Ibid.

Chapter 8: The Mind–Body Problem

p. 264 *antidepressants . . . in conjunction with CBT*: O'Malley, P. G., Jackson, J. L., Santoro, J., et al., 'Antidepressant therapy for unexplained symptoms and symptom syndromes', The Journal of Family Practice, 48.12 (1999) 980–90. https://pubmed.ncbi.nlm.nih.gov/10628579/

p. 264 *lack of a large-scale clinical trial*: Barsky, A. J., 'The patient with hypochondriasis', New England Journal of Medicine, 345.19 (2001) 1395–9. https://doi.org/10.1056/NEJMcp002896

p. 265 *come to different conclusions*: Spitzer, R. L., and Fleiss, J. L., 'A re-analysis of the reliability of psychiatric diagnosis', British Journal of Psychiatry, 125.587 (1974) 341–7. https://doi.org/10.1192/bjp.125.4.341

p. 266   *'When I touch your skin ...'*: Miller, W., 'Mind-Body Problem'

p. 268   *'immature defence'*: Vaillant, G. E., 'Involuntary coping mechanisms: a psychodynamic perspective', Dialogues in Clinical Neuroscience, 13.3 (2011) 366–70. https://doi.org/10.31887/DCNS.2011.13.2/gvaillant

p. 269   *'functional paralysis'*: Harris, W., *Nerve Injuries and Shock* (Oxford War Primers, 1915), preface

p. 269   *'The human response to psychological trauma ...'*: van der Kolk, B., 'Posttraumatic stress disorder and the nature of trauma', Dialogues in Clinical Neuroscience, 2.1 (2000) 7–22. https://doi.org/10.31887/DCNS.2000.2.1/bvdkolk

p. 269   *A large study of military veterans*: McFarlane Ao, A. C., and Graham, D. K., 'The ambivalence about accepting the prevalence somatic symptoms in PTSD: is PTSD a somatic disorder?', Journal of Psychiatric Research, 143 (2021) 388–94. https://doi.org/10.1016/j.jpsychires.2021.09.030

p. 270   *'more medical visits ...'*: Trickett, P. K., Noll, J. G., and Putnam, F. W., 'The impact of sexual abuse on female development: lessons from a multigenerational, longitudinal research study', Development and Psychopathology, 23.2 (2011) 453–76. https://doi.org/10.1017/S0954579411000174

p. 271   *the brain's smoke detector*: van der Kolk, B., *The Body Keeps the Score: Brain, Mind, and Body in the Healing of Trauma* (Penguin, 2015), p. 87

p. 273   *'Like a splinter ...'*: Ibid., p. 289

p. 273   *'adverse childhood experiences'*: Reiser, S. J., Power, H. A., and Wright, K. D., 'Examining the relationships between childhood abuse history, attachment, and health anxiety', Journal of Health Psychology, 26.7 (2021) 1085–95. https://doi.org/10.1177/1359105319869804

p. 273   *appraises their feelings of illness*: Traino, K. A., Espeleta, H. C., Dattilo, T. M., et al., 'Childhood adversity and illness appraisals as predictors of health anxiety in emerging adults with a chronic illness', Journal of Clinical Psychology in Medical Settings, 30 (2022) 143–52. https://doi.org/10.1007/s10880-022-09870-z

p. 276   *Some studies*: Shipley, G., Wilde, S., and Hudson, M., 'What do clients say about their experiences of eye movement desensitisation and reprocessing therapy? A systematic review of the literature', European Journal of Trauma & Dissociation, 6.2 (2022) 100226. https://doi.org/10.1016/j.ejtd.2021.100226

p. 276   *including van der Kolk's own*: van der Kolk, B., *The Body* . . ., p. 299

p. 276   '*conditionally recommends*': https://www.apa.org/ptsd-guideline/ treatments/eye-movement-reprocessing

p. 276   '*limited evidence*': https://www.nice.org.uk/guidance/ng116

p. 279   *In one account*: 'When chronic pain becomes who you are'. https:// slate.com/technology/2022/06/chronic-pain-identity-spoonies-support-recovery.html

p. 279   *women with endometriosis*: Marschall, H., Hansen, K. E., Forman, A., et al., 'Storying endometriosis: examining relationships between narrative identity, mental health, and pain', Journal of Research in Personality, 91 (2021) 104062. https://doi.org/10.1016/j.jrp.2020.104062

p. 280   *reduce their healthcare costs*: Louw, A., Zimney, K., Puentedura, E. J., et al., 'The efficacy of pain neuroscience education on musculoskeletal pain: a systematic review of the literature', Physiotherapy Theory and Practice, 32.5 (2016) 332–55. https:// doi.org/10.1080/09593985.2016.1194646

p. 282   *willing to be mortal*: Wilhelmsen, I., 'Hypochondriasis or health anxiety', in *Encyclopedia of Human Behavior* (Elsevier, 2012), pp. 385–91. https://doi.org/10.1016/B978-0-12-375000-6.00197-X

Select Bibliography

Introduction: The People Made of Glass

Belling, C., *A Condition of Doubt* (OUP, 2012)

Kolb, P. (ed.), *Marcel Proust: Selected Letters 1880–1903* (University of Chicago Press, 1983)

Ladee, G. A., *Hypochondriacal Syndromes* (Elsevier, 1966)

Lipsitt, D. R., and Starcevic. V. (eds.), *Hypochondriasis: Modern Perspectives on an Ancient Malady* (OUP, 2001)

Proust, M., *The Guermantes Way*, translation by Scott Moncrieff, C. K., and Kilmartin, T. (Modern Library, 2003)

Shepherd, V., *A History of Delusions: The Glass King, a Substitute Husband and a Walking Corpse* (Oneworld, 2022)

Speak, G., 'An odd kind of melancholy: reflections on the glass delusion in Europe (1440–1680)', *History of Psychiatry*, 1.2 (1990) 191–206

Chapter 1: The Origins of the Ancient Malady

Edwin Smith Surgical Papyrus

Kahun Gynaecological Papyrus

Bryan, C. P., and Smith, G. E., *Ancient Egyptian Medicine: The Papyrus Ebers* (Ares, 1930)

Geller, M. J., *Ancient Babylonian Medicine: Theory and Practice* (Wiley-Blackwell, 2010)

Ludlul bēl nēmeqi, Tablet 2, Line 50. Translation by Lambert, W. G., in *Babylonian Wisdom Literature* (Clarendon, 1960)

da Silva Veiga, P. A., *Health and Medicine in Ancient Egypt: Magic and Science* (University of Michigan Press, 2009)

Chapter 2: All Disease Begins in the Gut

Aphorisms Of Hippocrates, translation by Marks, E. (Collins, 1817)

Hippocrates, *Epidemics II*

Plato, *Timaeus*

Arikha, N., *Passions and Tempers: A History of the Humors* (Ecco, 2007)

Capra, F., *The Turning Point: Science, Society, and the Rising Culture* (Bantam Books, 1983)

Nuland, S. B., *Doctors: The Biography of Medicine* (Knopf, 2011)

Pormann, P. E., *Rufus of Ephesus On Melancholy* (Mohr Siebeck, 2008)

Chapter 3: Sharp Belchings and Windy Melancholy

Armstrong, J. K., *Seinfeldia* (Simon & Schuster, 2017)

Bloom, C., *Leaving a Doll's House* (Virago Press, 1996)

Boswell, J., *Life of Dr Johnson* (1791)

Burton, R. and Gowland, A. (ed.), *The Anatomy of Melancholy* (Penguin, 2023)

Donne, J., *Devotions Upon Emergent Occasions* (Knopf, 1999)

Donne, J., *The Major Works* (OUP, 2008)

Lund, M. A., *A User's Guide to Melancholy* (CUP, 2021)

Matthews, B., *Molière: His Life and His Works* (Hardpress, 2013)

Radden, J., *Melancholic Habits* (OUP, 2016)

Roth, P., *The Counterlife* (Vintage, 2005)

Rundell, K., *Super-Infinite: The Transformations of John Donne* (Faber, 2022)

Scarry, E. (ed.), *Literature and the Body: Essays on Populations and Persons* (Johns Hopkins University Press, 1990)

Chapter 4: Spirits, Vapours and Nerves

Arnaud, S., *On Hysteria: The Invention of a Medical Category Between 1670 and 1820* (University of Chicago Press, 2015)

Baur, S., *Hypochondria: Woeful Imaginings* (University of California Press, 1988)

Foucault, M., *Madness and Civilization: A History of Insanity in the Age of Reason*, translation by Howard, R. (Vintage Books, 1988)

Gilman, C. P., *The Living of Charlotte Perkins Gilman: An Autobiography* (University of Wisconsin Press, 1990)

Gilman, C. P., *The Yellow Wallpaper and Selected Writings* (Little, Brown, 2009)

Gilman, S. L., King, H., Porter, R., et al., *Hysteria Beyond Freud* (University of California Press, 1993)

Scull, A., *Hysteria: The Biography* (Oxford University Press, 2009)

Chapter 5: The Rise and Rise of the Quack

Benedetti, F., *Placebo Effects: Understanding the Mechanisms in Health and Disease* (Oxford University Press, 2009)

Brent-Dyer, E. M., *The School at the Chalet* (Armada, 1994)

Carreyrou, J., *Bad Blood: Secrets and Lies in a Silicon Valley Startup* (Picador, 2019)

Curth, L. H., ed., *From Physick to Pharmacology: Five Hundred Years of British Drug Retailing* (Routledge, 2017)

Day, C. A., *Consumptive Chic: A History of Beauty, Fashion, and Disease* (Bloomsbury, 2017)

Dillon, B., *Tormented Hope* (Penguin, 2009)

Grinnell, G. C., *The Age of Hypochondria: Interpreting Romantic Health and Illness* (Palgrave Macmillan, 2010)

Jameson, E., *A Natural History of Quackery* (Michael Joseph, 1961)

Porter, R. (ed.). *George Cheyne: The English Malady* (1733), Tavistock Classics in the History of Psychiatry (Tavistock/Routledge, 1991)

Porter, R. *Quacks* (Routledge, 2000)

Rousseau, G. S., *Nervous Acts: Essays on Literature, Culture and Sensibility* (Palgrave Macmillan, 2004)

Shorter, C. K., *The Brontës Life and Letters Vol II* (Hodder and Stoughton, 1908)

Strathern, P., *Quacks, Rogues and Charlatans of the RCP* (Little Brown, 2016)

Chapter 6: All in My Head

Bartlett, N., *Jane Austen: Reflections of a Reader* (OBP, 2021)

Boyer, A., *The Undying* (Allen Lane, 2019)

Charon, R., 'Narrative medicine: a model for empathy,

reflection, profession, and trust', *Journal of the American Medical Association*, 286.15 (2001)

Charon, R., *Narrative Medicine* (OUP, 2008)

Frank, A. W., *The Wounded Storyteller: Body, Illness, and Ethics* (University of Chicago Press, 2006)

Freud, S., *A General Introduction to Psychoanalysis* (Boni & Liveright, 1920)

Freud, S., *The Complete Letters of Sigmund Freud to Wilhelm Fliess, 1887–1904*, translation by Masson, J. M. (Belknap Press. 1986)

Khakpour, P., *Sick* (Canongate, 2018)

Larkin, P., *Required Writing: Miscellaneous Pieces 1955–1982* (Farrar Straus Giroux, 1984)

Larkin, P., *Whitsun Weddings* (Faber, 1964)

Moser, B., *Sontag: Her Life* (Penguin, 2020)

Motion, A., *Philip Larkin: A Writer's Life* (Gardners Books, 1994)

Sontag, S., *Illness as Metaphor* (Penguin, 2009)

Starcevic, V., and Noyes Jr., R. *Hypochondriasis and Health Anxiety: A Guide for Clinicians* (OUP, 2014)

Tomalin, C., *Jane Austen: A Life* (Penguin, 2012)

Woolf, V., *A Writer's Diary* (Persephone Books, 2012)

Woolf, V., *Selected Essays* (OUP, 2009)

Chapter 7: We Know Too Much

Green, J., *The Anthropocene Reviewed* (Dutton, 2021)

Jamison, L., *The Recovering* (Granta, 2018)

Jerome, J. K., *Three Men in a Boat* (OUP, 2008)

Luparello, T., Lyons, H. A., Bleecker, E. R., et al., 'Influences of suggestion on airway reactivity in asthmatic subjects', *Psychosomatic Medicine*, 30.6 (1968) 819–25

Montague, J., *The Imaginary Patient* (Granta, 2022)
O'Connell, J., *I Told You I Was Ill: Adventures in Hypochondria* (Short Books, 2006)
Risse, G. B., *Mending Bodies, Saving Souls: A History of Hospitals* (Oxford University Press, 1999)

Chapter 8: The Mind–Body Problem

Autton, N., *Pain: An Exploration* (Darton, Longman & Todd, 1986)
Boyle, E., *Fierce Appetites* (Sandycove, 2022)
van der Kolk, B., *The Body Keeps the Score: Brain, Mind, and Body in the Healing of Trauma* (Penguin, 2015)
Shapiro, F., *Eye Movement Desensitization and Reprocessing (EMDR) Therapy: Basic Principles, Protocols, and Procedures* (Guildford Press, 2018)
Wang, E. W., *The Collected Schizophrenias* (Penguin, 2019)

Acknowledgements

Without the support and patience of my agent Sophie Lambert over the more than five years it has taken me to bring this book into being, I would not be writing this now. Her expert assistance, along with that of my US agent Amelia Atlas, has been invaluable in shaping this idea into something that I hope readers can find solace and comfort in.

My editor at Granta, Laura Barber, instantly understood what I wanted this book to be and has made it better at every step of the way. I couldn't imagine a better collaborator. Sarah Murphy and Helen Atsma, my editors at Ecco in the US, have also helped me greatly in bringing the best out of the subject, and I am indebted to them all for such a smooth and organised editorial process. I am very much obliged, too, to the talented teams at both publishers who have lent their expertise to producing a book of which I'm very proud.

I would like to thank staff at the following institutions for their assistance during my research: Bebington Central Library, the Bodleian Library, the British Library, the London Library, Gladstone's Library, Liverpool Central Library and the Wellcome Collection. In addition, Professor Mark Geller and Professor Maria Grazia Masetti-Rouault generously provided expertise in Babylonian literature and cuneiform texts, for which I am very grateful.

To everyone who has taken the time to speak to me about their experiences of hypochondria: thank you. I know it wasn't easy to do.

Uri Bram, Robert Cottrell and Sylvia Bishop of The Browser have been the most generous of colleagues and I am forever grateful that I get to work with them. Likewise, I am thankful for the help of Leandra Griffith and Euan McAleece, who keep my podcast running even when I am distracted by other projects.

I would like to thank my parents, Des and Terry Crampton, and my sister Steph. I am also grateful to the following people for their advice along the way: Dan Bloom, Kat Brown, Jonn Elledge, Cal Flyn, Lilith Johnstone, Helen Lewis, Elizabeth Minkel, Jenni Munroe, Samira Shackle, Barbara Smith and Helen Zaltzman.

The existence of this book owes a great deal to the presence of Morris the Clumber spaniel in my life. His cheerfulness and need for regular walks are essential on bad writing days. My biggest debt of gratitude is to my beloved husband Guy, to whom this book is dedicated. He always believed I could do this even when I did my best to convince him otherwise. Thank you.

Index